Stahl's Illustrated

Treatments for Mood Disorders

Stephen M Stahl, MD, PhD is Professor of Psychiatry and Neuroscience at UC Riverside and at UC San Diego, Honorary Visiting Senior Fellow, University of Cambridge, UK, and Chairman of the Neuroscience Education Institute, Carlsbad.

Stahl's Illustrated

Treatments for Mood Disorders

Stephen M. Stahl
University of California, San Diego

Sabrina K. Segal
Neuroscience Education Institute

Nancy Muntner
Illustrations

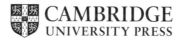

COPYRIGHT

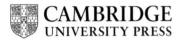
CAMBRIDGE
UNIVERSITY PRESS

Shaftesbury Road, Cambridge CB2 8EA, United Kingdom
One Liberty Plaza, 20th Floor, New York, NY 10006, USA
477 Williamstown Road, Port Melbourne, VIC 3207, Australia
314–321, 3rd Floor, Plot 3, Splendor Forum, Jasola District Centre, New Delhi – 110025, India
103 Penang Road, #05-06/07, Visioncrest Commercial, Singapore 238467

Cambridge University Press is part of Cambridge University Press & Assessment,
a department of the University of Cambridge.

We share the University's mission to contribute to society through the pursuit of
education, learning and research at the highest international levels of excellence.

www.cambridge.org
Information on this title: www.cambridge.org/9781009009119
DOI: 10.1017/9781009003377

© Cambridge University Press and Assessment 2023

First published 2023

Printed in Mexico by Litográfica Ingramex, S.A. de C.V.

A catalogue record for this publication is available from the British Library

ISBN 978-1-009-00911-9 Paperback

Cambridge University Press & Assessment has no responsibility for the persistence
or accuracy of URLs for external or third-party internet websites referred to in this
publication and does not guarantee that any content on such websites is, or will
remain, accurate or appropriate.

Every effort has been made in preparing this book to provide accurate and
up-to-date information that is in accord with accepted standards and practice
at the time of publication. Although case histories are drawn from actual cases,
every effort has been made to disguise the identities of the individuals involved.
Nevertheless, the authors, editors, and publishers can make no warranties that the
information contained herein is totally free from error, not least because clinical
standards are constantly changing through research and regulation. The authors,
editors, and publishers therefore disclaim all liability for direct or consequential
damages resulting from the use of material contained in this book. Readers
are strongly advised to pay careful attention to information provided by the
manufacturer of any drugs or equipment that they plan to use.

PREFACE

These books are designed to be fun, with all concepts illustrated by full-color images and the text serving as a supplement to figures, images, and tables. The visual learner will find that this book makes psychopharmacological concepts easy to master, while the non-visual learner may enjoy a shortened text version of complex psychopharmacological concepts. Each chapter builds upon previous chapters, synthesizing information from basic biology and diagnostics to building treatment plans and dealing with complications and comorbidities.

Novices may want to approach this book by first looking through all the graphics, gaining a feel for the visual vocabulary on which our psychopharmacological concepts rely. After this once-over glance, we suggest going back through the book to incorporate the images with supporting text. Learning from visual concepts and textual supplements should reinforce one another, providing you with solid conceptual understanding at each step along the way.

Readers more familiar with these topics should find that going back and forth between images and text provides an interaction with which to vividly conceptualize complex psychopharmacology. You may find yourself using this book frequently to refresh your psychopharmacological knowledge. And you will hopefully refer your colleagues to this desk reference.

This book is intended as a conceptual overview of different topics; we provide you with a visual-based language to incorporate the rules of psychopharmacology at the expense of discussing the exceptions to these rules. The References section at the end gives you a good start for more in-depth learning about particular concepts presented here. *Stahl's Essential Psychopharmacology* and *Stahl's Essential Psychopharmacology: The Prescriber's Guide* can be helpful supplementary tools for more in-depth information on particular topics in this book. You can also search topics in psychopharmacology on the Neuroscience Education Institute's website (www.neiglobal.com) for lectures, courses, slides, and related articles.

Whether you are a novice or an experienced psychopharmacologist, this book will hopefully lead you to think critically about the complexities involved in psychiatric disorders and their treatments.

Best wishes for your educational journey into the fascinating field of psychopharmacology!

Stephen M. Stahl

Table of Contents

CME/CE Information

Released: September 1, 2022
CME/CE credit expires: September 1, 2025

Target Audience: This activity has been developed for the entire healthcare team specializing in mental health and includes education for nurse practitioners, physicians, psychologists, physician assistants, pharmacists, and social workers. All other mental healthcare team members interested in psychopharmacology are welcome for advanced study.

Learning Objectives: After completing this activity, you should be better able to:

- Identify the neurobiology of malfunctioning circuits that underlie the spectrum of mood disorder symptoms
- Implement evidence-based treatments that target malfunctioning neurocircuitry in mood disorders
- Recognize novel therapeutic approaches and pharmacological targets in development for the treatment of mood disorders

Accreditation: In support of improving patient care, Neuroscience Education Institute (NEI) is jointly accredited by the Accreditation Council for Continuing Medical Education (ACCME), the Accreditation Council for Pharmacy Education (ACPE), and the American Nurses Credentialing Center (ANCC), to provide continuing education for the healthcare team.

NEI designates this enduring material for a maximum of 10.0 *AMA PRA Category 1 Credits*™. Physicians should claim only the credit commensurate with the extent of their participation in the activity.

The content in this activity pertaining to pharmacology is worth 10.0 continuing education hours of pharmacotherapeutics.

Credit Types: The following are being offered for this activity:

- Nurse Practitioner: ANCC contact hours
- Pharmacy: ACPE application-based contact hours
- Physician: ACCME *AMA PRA Category 1 Credits*™
- Physician Assistant: AAPA Category 1 CME credits
- Psychology: APA CE credits
- Social Work: ASWB-ACE CE credits

- Non-Physician Member of the Mental Healthcare Team: Certificate of Participation stating the program is designated for *AMA PRA Category 1 Credits*™

Optional Posttest and CME/CE Credit: The optional posttest with CME/CE credits is available online for a fee (waived for NEI Members). A posttest score of 70% or higher is required to receive credit. Go to: https://nei.global/22-Stahl-illus-mood

Peer Review: The content was peer-reviewed by a PhD with a background in neuropharmacology and mood disorders to ensure the scientific accuracy and medical relevance of information presented and its independence from bias. NEI takes responsibility for the content, quality, and scientific integrity of this CME activity.

Disclosures: All individuals in a position to influence or control content are required to disclose all relevant financial relationships. Potential conflicts were identified and mitigated prior to the activity being planned, developed, or presented.

Author
Sabrina K. Bradbury-Segal, PhD
Medical Writer, Neuroscience Education Institute, Carlsbad, CA
No financial relationships to disclose.

Editor
Stephen M. Stahl, MD, PhD, DSc (Hon.)
Clinical Professor, Department of Psychiatry and Neuroscience, University of California, Riverside School of Medicine, Riverside, CA
Adjunct Professor, Department of Psychiatry, University of California, San Diego School of Medicine, La Jolla, CA
Honorary Visiting Senior Fellow, University of Cambridge, Cambridge, UK
Editor-in-Chief, CNS Spectrums
Director of Psychopharmacology Services, California Department of State Hospitals, Sacramento, CA
Grant/Research: Acadia, Alkermes, Allergan/AbbVie, Arbor, AssureX, AstraZeneca, Avanir, Axovant, Biogen, Braeburn, BristolMyer Squibb, Celgene, CeNeRex, Cephalon, Dey, Eisai, Forest, GenOmind, Glaxo Smith Kline, Harmony Biosciences, Indivior, Intra-Cellular, Ironshore, Janssen, JayMac, Jazz, Lilly, Lundbeck, Merck, Neurocrine, Neuronetics, Novartis, Otsuka, Pear, Pfizer, Reviva, Roche, Sage, Servier, Shire, Sprout, Sunovion, Supernus, Takeda, Teva, Tonix, Torrent, Vanda
Consultant/Advisor: Acadia, Adamas, Alkermes, Allergan/AbbVie, Arbor,

AstraZeneca, Avanir, Axovant, Axsome, Biogen, Biomarin, Biopharma, Celgene, ClearView, Concert, DepotMed, EMD Serono, Eisai, Eurolink, Ferring, Forest, Genomind, Innovative Science Solutions, Impel, Intra-Cellular, Ironshore, Janssen, Jazz, Karuna, Lilly, Lundbeck, Merck, Neos, Neurocrine, NeuroPharma, Novartis, Noveida, Otsuka, Perrigo, Pfizer, Pierre Fabre, Proxymm, Relmada, Reviva, Sage, Servier, Shire, Sprout, Sunovion, Takeda, Taliaz, Teva, Tonix, Tris, Trius, Vanda, Vertex, Viforpharma

Speakers Bureau: Acadia, Genentech, Janssen, Lundbeck, Merck, Otsuka, Servier, Sunovion, Takeda, Teva

Board Member: Genomind, RCT Logic

Options Holdings: Delix, Genomind, Lipidio

The **Planning Committee**, **Content Editor**, **Design Staff**, and **Peer Reviewer** have no financial relationships to disclose.

Disclosure of Off-Label Use: This educational activity may include discussion of unlabeled and/or investigational uses of agents that are not currently labeled for such use by the FDA. Please consult the product prescribing information for full disclosure of labeled uses.

Cultural Linguistic Competency and Implicit Bias: A variety of resources addressing cultural and linguistic competency and strategies for understanding and reducing implicit bias can be found at: https://nei.global/CLC-IB-handout

Support: This activity is supported solely by the provider, NEI.

Mood disorders involve symptoms that extend far beyond disruption of mood, rendering them challenging to diagnose, monitor, and treat. An estimated 21.4% of adults in the United States experience a mood disorder at some point in their lives (Kessler et al., 2007). Annually, an estimated 21 million (8.4%) Americans are diagnosed with major depressive disorder (MDD), and an estimated 7 million (2.8%) are diagnosed with bipolar disorder (BP) (SAMHSA, 2021). The classic perspective of mood disorders has been to view mood symptoms of mania and depression as distinct and opposite "poles." As our understanding of mood disorders expands, it is becoming increasingly apparent that mood disorders exist along a continuum or spectrum and do not operate as distinct "poles." This has important implications for clinical management and treatment of mood disorders.

In the following pages, we will describe the spectrum of symptoms included in mood disorders, the neurocircuitry that underlies those symptoms, and the evidence-based therapeutic targets for the treatment of those symptoms. We will also address best practices for early screening/detection and long-term management/treatment of mood disorders. Chapters 1–2 describe the neurobiological models and neurocircuitry that underlie various mood disorders and how malfunctioning circuits are connected to symptoms. Chapters 3–4 describe the mechanisms that underlie evidence-based treatments and how they can improve neurocircuitry in mood disorders, even in treatment resistance. Chapters 5–6 examine advancements in the development of novel evidence-based pharmacological treatments, and the use of nonpharmacological methods as adjunctive treatments or standalone treatments for depressive disorders.

Classification and Symptoms of Mood Disorders and Disease Models of Depressive Disorders

Mood disorders are often referred to as affective disorders. Affect is the external display of emotion, while emotion that is felt internally is referred to as mood. Disorders of mood consist of a variety of symptoms that extend beyond disruption of mood. The most effective clinical approach to treatment is to first construct a diagnosis from an individual patient's symptoms profile, and then deconstruct its component symptoms so that each symptom can be addressed individually as a therapeutic target. A neurobiological approach to treatment begins with matching each symptom to its hypothetically malfunctioning brain circuit, regulated by one or more neurotransmitters. Drug selection should then target specific neurotransmitters in the symptomatic brain circuits in the individual patient. Targeting these malfunctioning circuits and improving neural processing should result in reduced symptoms.

Traditionally, mood symptoms of mania and depression have been considered as being "poles" apart. Patients who experience just the down or depressive pole are classified as having unipolar depression. Patients who at different times experience the up (mania or hypomania) pole and the down pole (depressive pole) are classified as having bipolar disorder. Bipolar I disorder is characterized by full-blown manic episodes typically followed by depressive episodes. Bipolar II disorder is characterized by at least one hypomanic episode and one major depressive episode. Finally, depression and mania may even occur simultaneously, which is classified as a "mixed" mood state or "mixed features" according to the *Diagnostic and Statistical Manual of Mental Disorders Fifth Ed. Text Revision (DSM-5-TR)*. The introduction of the mixed features modifier has moved the field away from considering depression and mania as distinct categories and towards the concept that they are opposite ends of the spectrum.

The Mood Disorder Spectrum

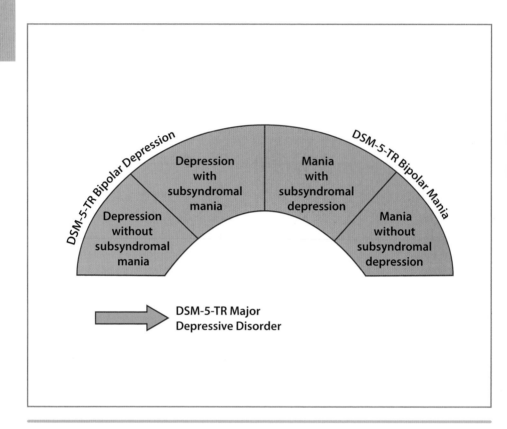

FIGURE 1.1. The field has moved away from characterizing depression and mania as distinct categories and now views them as opposite ends of a spectrum, with varying degrees of either or both between. Many patients are not purely manic or depressed, but rather they experience a mixture of symptoms. The specific mix of mood symptoms may change along the mood spectrum over the course of the illness (Stahl, 2021).

Description of Depressive State Symptoms in Mood Disorders

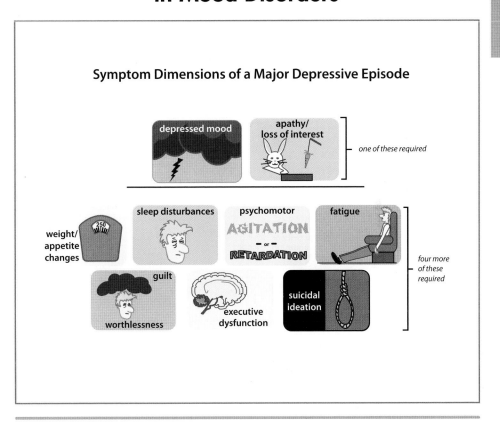

FIGURE 1.2. According to the DSM-5-TR (American Psychiatric Association, 2022), a major depressive episode is characterized by either depressed mood or loss of interest and at least four of the following: fatigue, insomnia/hypersomnia, weight/appetite alterations, fatigue, psychomotor agitation/retardation, feelings of guilt or worthlessness, executive dysfunction, and suicidal ideation (Stahl, 2021).

Description of Manic State Symptoms in Mood Disorders

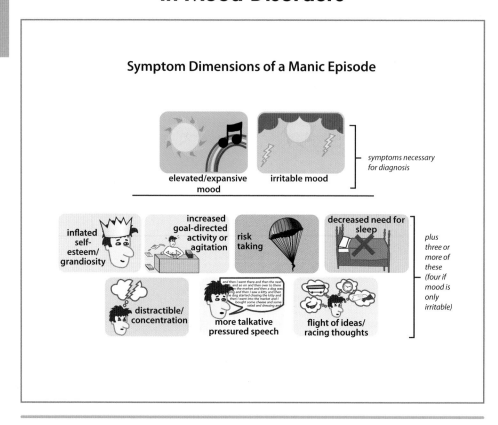

FIGURE 1.3. According to the DSM-5-TR, a manic episode consists of either expansive/ elevated mood or irritable mood and at least three of the following (four if mood is irritable): increased goal-directed activity or agitation, inflated self-esteem/grandiosity, decreased need for sleep, risk taking, distractibility, racing thoughts, and pressured speech (Stahl, 2021).

The Spectrum of Mood Disorder Symptoms

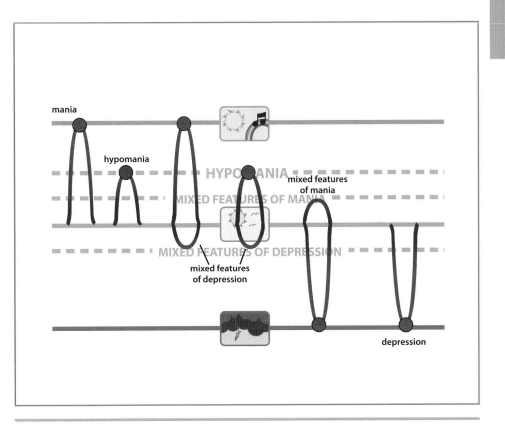

FIGURE 1.4. Mood disorder symptoms occur along a spectrum, with the polar ends consisting of pure mania or hypomania (the "up" pole) and pure depression (the "down" pole). Patients can also experience simultaneous symptoms of both poles. This is referred to as mania/hypomania with mixed features of depression, or depression with mixed features of mania. Patients may experience any combination of these symptoms over the course of the illness. Subsyndromal manic or depressive episodes may also occur, in which case there are not enough symptoms or the symptoms are not severe enough to fit the diagnostic criteria for one of these episodes. The presentation of mood disorders can vary widely, both between individuals and within the individual patient (Stahl, 2021).

Mixed Features of Manic, Hypomanic, and Major Depressive Episodes

Manic or hypomanic episode, with mixed features
Full criteria for manic or hypomanic episode
At least three of the following symptoms of depression:
Depressed mood
Loss of interest or pleasure
Psychomotor retardation
Fatigue or loss of energy
Feelings of worthlessness or excessive or inappropriate guilt
Recurrent thoughts of death or suicidal ideation/actions
Depressive episode, with mixed features
Full criteria for a major depressive episode
At least three of the following manic/hypomanic symptoms:
Elevated, expansive mood (e.g., feeling high, excited, or hyper)
Inflated self-esteem or grandiosity
More talkative than usual or feeling pressured to keep talking
Flight of ideas or subjective experience that thoughts are racing
Increase in energy or goal-directed activity
Increased or excessive involvement in activities that have a high potential for painful consequences
Decreased need for sleep
(*Not included: psychomotor agitation)
(*Not included: irritability)
(*Not included: distractibility)

FIGURE 1.5. When screening for mania/hypomania with mixed features, the patient's symptoms must meet the full criteria for mania and at least three of the depressive symptoms listed in this chart. When screening for depression with mixed features, the symptoms must meet full criteria for a depressive episode, along with at least three of the manic/hypomanic symptoms listed in this chart. When screening for depression with mixed features, assessing whether there is a family history of mania or hypomania should be highly prioritized (Stahl, 2021; Stahl and Morrisette, 2019).

Identifying Depression Within the Mood Disorder Spectrum

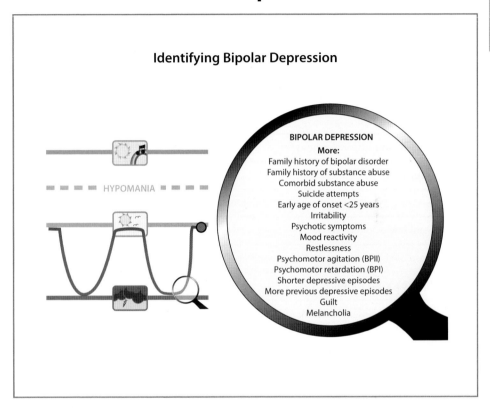

Identifying Bipolar Depression

HYPOMANIA

BIPOLAR DEPRESSION
More:
Family history of bipolar disorder
Family history of substance abuse
Comorbid substance abuse
Suicide attempts
Early age of onset <25 years
Irritability
Psychotic symptoms
Mood reactivity
Restlessness
Psychomotor agitation (BPII)
Psychomotor retardation (BPI)
Shorter depressive episodes
More previous depressive episodes
Guilt
Melancholia

FIGURE 1.6. Aside from a history of prior manic/hypomanic episodes, patients with bipolar depression are diagnosed with identical criteria as patients with unipolar depression. While they may have similar symptoms, the long-term outcomes differ between patients with bipolar depression versus unipolar depression, thus treatment approaches are different. The wrong treatment approach could have debilitating effects on the patient's quality of life and missed or delayed diagnosis is common. Over one-third of patients with unipolar depression are subsequently re-diagnosed with bipolar disorder and up to 60% of depressed patients with bipolar II disorder are initially diagnosed with unipolar depression. Reasons for missed or delayed diagnosis may be that the patient has either not experienced mania/hypomania yet or that prior occurrence was missed at screening (Stahl, 2021).

Distinguishing Unipolar Depression From Bipolar Depression

Who's your Daddy?
What is your family history of:
• mood disorder?
• psychiatric hospitalizations?
• suicide?
• anyone who took lithium, mood stabilizers, drugs for psychosis or depression?
• anyone who received ECT?
These can be indications of a unipolar or bipolar spectrum disorder in relatives.
Where's your Mama?
I need to get additional history about you from someone close to you, such as your mother or your spouse.
Patients may especially lack insight about their manic symptoms and underreport them.

FIGURE 1.7. While it is important to distinguish bipolar depression from unipolar depression, it can be challenging while the patient is in the depressed state. There are two main questions that can help to determine whether a patient is unipolar or bipolar: "Who's your daddy?" and "Where's your mama?" The first question, "Who's your daddy?" equates to taking a family history. A first-degree relative with a bipolar spectrum disorder increases the chance that the patient has bipolar depression versus unipolar depression, and it is arguably the most robust and reliable risk factor for bipolar depression. The second question "Where's your mama?" equates to collecting additional history from someone who is close to the patient (e.g., roommate, caretaker, spouse, family member). This question is important because many patients with bipolar depression underreport their manic symptoms (Stahl, 2021). ECT, electroconvulsive therapy.

Is Major Depressive Disorder Progressive?

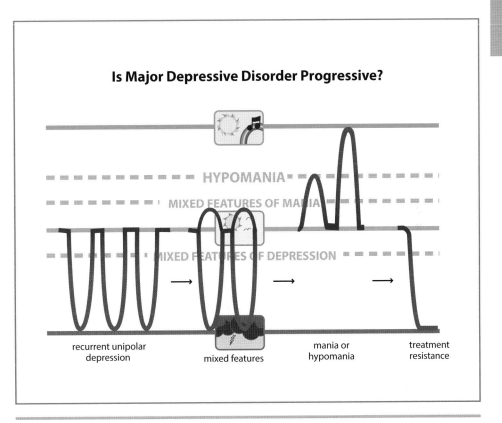

FIGURE 1.8. There is evidence that mood disorders may be progressive. While screening and monitoring patients with mood disorders it is essential to look for mixed features in depressed patients, whether they have unipolar or bipolar depression. There is evidence that unipolar depression can progress to mixed features, mixed features can progress to bipolar disorder, and bipolar disorder can progress to treatment resistance. Even subthreshold manic symptoms are strongly associated with conversion to bipolar disorder, with each manic symptom increasing the risk by 30%. Approximately one-quarter of adult patients with unipolar depression and about one-third of all patients with bipolar I or II depression have subsyndromal symptoms of mania, and there are even higher estimates of mixed features in children and adolescents with unipolar depression. Early detection and treatment of all symptoms, whether manic or depressive, may prevent the progression of the mood disorder (Fiedorowicz et al., 2011).

Evolving Disease Models in Depressive Disorders

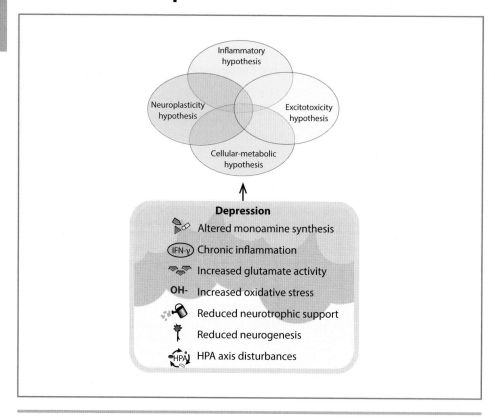

FIGURE 1.9. There is a growing body of research on the pathogenesis of depression identifying interactions between multiple biological systems. The major disease models are centered around altered monoamine functioning, chronic inflammation, excitotoxicity, neurogenesis and neuroplasticity disruptions/reduced neurotrophic support, endocrine problems, and cellular-metabolic factors (Dowlati et al., 2010; Howren et al., 2009; Miller et al., 2009; Pace et al., 2007; Pariante, 2009). As our understanding grows about the integration of these models, and how they are influenced by external/environmental factors, the more useful they will become to the screening and treatment of depressive disorders. It is important to remember that multiple components from these various models may be contributing to depressive symptoms and thus should be factored into the treatment plan for each individual patient. HPA, hypothalamic-pituitary-adrenal.

Early Disease Model in Depression: Monoamine Hypothesis

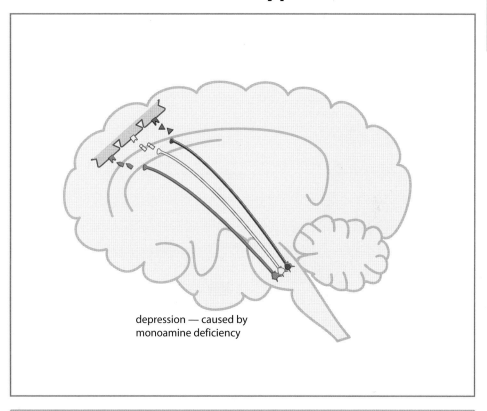

depression — caused by
monoamine deficiency

FIGURE 1.10. The classic neurobiological theory about the etiology of depression proposes that depressive disorders are caused by a deficiency of monoamine neurotransmission. It hypothesizes that the opposite, an excess of monoamine neurotransmission, causes mania. While mood disorders often involve dysfunction of one or more of these three monoamine systems (dopamine, serotonin, and norepinephrine), this "chemical imbalance" theory is now considered outdated and inaccurate, considering the lack of direct evidence to support it (Kohler et al., 2016; Stahl, 2021).

The Monoamine Receptor Hypothesis and Neurotrophic Factors

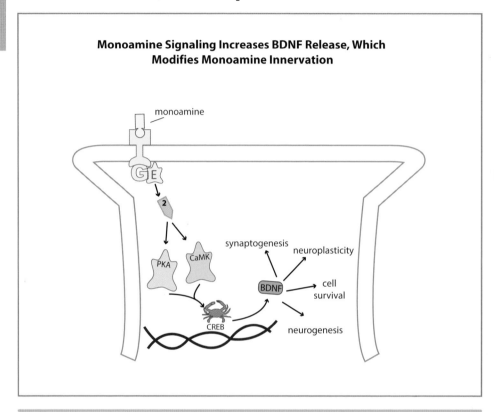

Monoamine Signaling Increases BDNF Release, Which Modifies Monoamine Innervation

FIGURE 1.11. While classic antidepressants result in increased levels of monoamines almost immediately after administration, the clinical improvement in depressive symptoms is not observed for weeks. Improved symptoms instead seem to correspond with downstream synthesis of growth factors such as brain-derived neurotrophic factor (BDNF). BDNF promotes the growth and development of young neurons, including monoaminergic neurons. It also enhances the survival of adult neurons and increases synaptogenesis. Monoamines can increase BDNF levels by initiating signal transduction cascades that result in its release. Thus, increased levels of monoamines that result from monoamine reuptake inhibitors may lead to downstream increases in neurotrophic factors, which correlates with the timeline of clinical improvement (Grady and Stahl, 2015; Stahl, 2021).

Beyond Monoamines: The Neuroplasticity Hypothesis of Depression

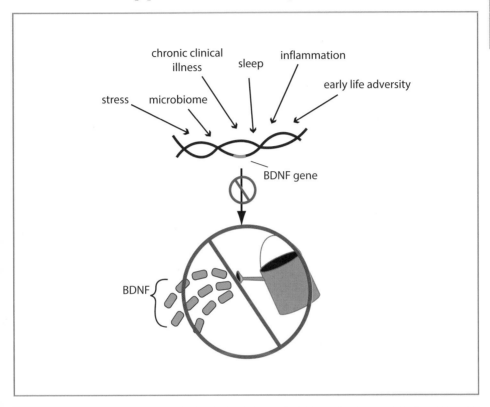

FIGURE 1.12. Environmental and genetic factors such as chronic illness, early life adversity, and alterations in the microbiome, stress, altered sleep, and inflammation may lead to the loss of growth factors, such as BDNF. Neurotrophic factors like BDNF are important to neuronal growth and survival, neuronal connections, and ultimately neuroplasticity. Genetic and environmental factors may contribute to neuroprogression in depression by resulting in epigenetic alterations that turn off genes for BDNF, reducing its production (Grady and Stahl, 2015; Stahl, 2021).

The Neuroprogression Hypothesis of Depression: Suppressed Brain-Derived Neurotrophic Factor

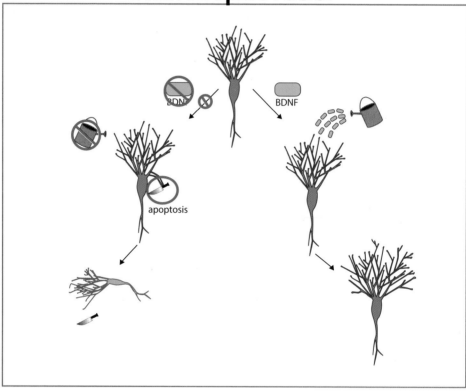

FIGURE 1.13. Suppression of BDNF results in a lack of synaptic maintenance, which in turn leads to a loss of synapses and dendritic arborization, ultimately resulting in apoptosis, or neuron cell death. This has been observed in structural magnetic resonance imaging studies of hippocampal volume, in which patients with depression have fewer dendritic spines. Abnormal functional neuroimaging (fMRI) studies of connectivity of brain circuits in depressed patients have also been reported (Grady and Stahl, 2015; Stahl, 2021).

The Neuroprogression Hypothesis in Depression

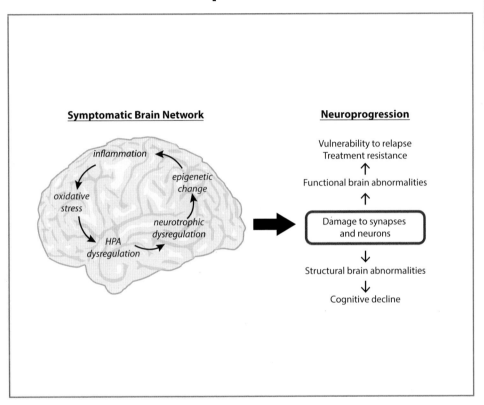

FIGURE 1.14. The neurobiological theory of neuroprogression is multifactorial. Neuroprogression in depression may be related to multiple interacting factors. Inflammation, dysregulation of the hypothalamic-pituitary-adrenal (HPA) axis, and oxidative stress may all influence neurotrophic dysregulation, resulting in epigenetic alterations that may further exacerbate inflammation, HPA axis dysfunction, and oxidative stress in a reciprocal fashion. Ultimately, all of these factors may contribute to the decrease in neurotrophic factors, the loss of synaptic connections, and the damage to neurons that may result in structural and functional brain abnormalities associated with depression (Stahl, 2021; Vavakova et al., 2015).

The Hypothalamic-Pituitary-Adrenal (HPA) Axis

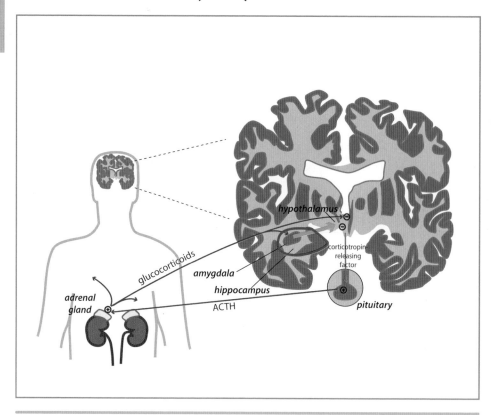

FIGURE 1.15. The normal stress response involves activation of the hypothalamus, resulting in increased corticotropin-releasing factor (CRF), which stimulates the release of adrenocorticotropic hormone (ACTH) from the pituitary gland. The release of ACTH causes the adrenal glands to secrete glucocorticoids, resulting in negative feedback to the hypothalamus, and inhibits the release of CRF, terminating the stress response. The HPA axis is also suppressed via input from the amygdala and hippocampus (Keller et al., 2017; Stahl, 2021).

Hippocampal Atrophy and Hyperactive HPA in Depression

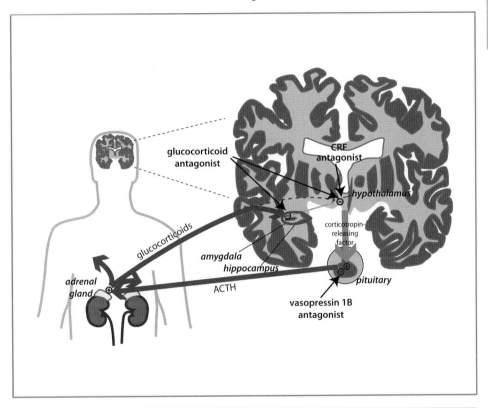

FIGURE 1.16. Neurons from the hippocampus and the amygdala normally suppress the HPA axis; thus, if chronic stress causes atrophy of hippocampal and amygdala neurons, the result could be overactivity of the HPA axis. Abnormalities of the HPA axis in depressed individuals have been reported, including reduction of negative feedback that inhibits the HPA axis, and elevated glucocorticoids. There is some evidence to suggest that high levels of glucocorticoids could be toxic to neurons. Novel antidepressant treatments that target CRF receptors and glucocorticoids are in testing (Keller et al., 2017; Stahl, 2021).

Neuroinflammation in Depression

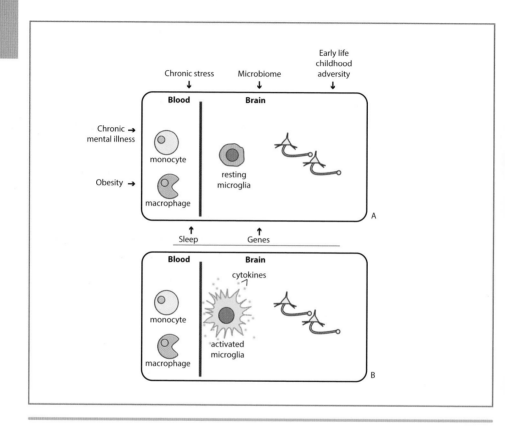

FIGURE 1.17. A) Chronic stress, early life adversity, obesity, chronic inflammatory diseases, long-term sleep disturbances, and disruption of the microbiome may all contribute to the development of neuroinflammation. B) When microglia become activated in the brain, due to these factors they can release proinflammatory cytokines (Brites and Fernandes, 2015; Stahl, 2021).

Neuroinflammation in Depression: Microglia and Proinflammatory Cytokines

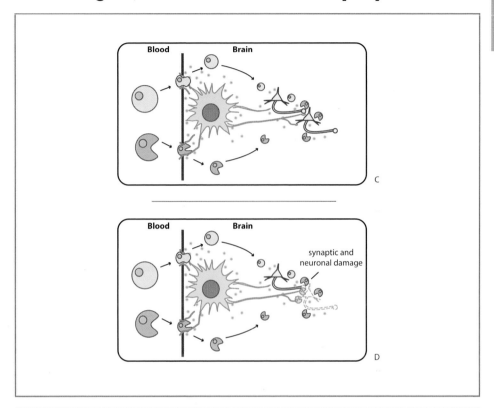

FIGURE 1.18. C) Proinflammatory cytokines attract immune cells, such as monocytes and macrophages, into the brain D) where they cause oxidative stress, HPA-dysfunction, reduction of growth factors like BDNF, and disruption of neurotransmission, and alter epigenetics to express unwanted genes that result in synaptic and neuronal damage (Brites and Fernandes, 2015; Stahl, 2021).

Circadian Rhythm Hypothesis in Depression

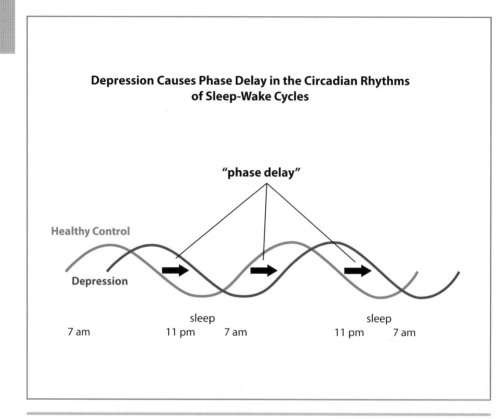

Depression Causes Phase Delay in the Circadian Rhythms of Sleep-Wake Cycles

FIGURE 1.19. Another neurobiological model suggests that depression is a circadian rhythm disorder that causes a phase delay in the sleep/wakefulness cycle. In patients with depression, the circadian rhythm is often "phase delayed," meaning that wakefulness is not promoted in the morning, so patients fall asleep later. They also have difficulty falling asleep, so this results in daytime sleepiness. The extent of this phase delay is correlated with the severity of the depression. Desynchronization of biological processes, such as circadian rhythms, can be pervasive in depression. There are genes referred to as clock genes that are sensitive to light-dark and operate in a circadian manner. Abnormalities in various clock genes have been associated with mood disorders. For patients with a circadian rhythm disorder, treatments such as bright light therapy, melatonin, and sleep deprivation can have therapeutic effects (Satyanarayanan et al., 2018; Stahl, 2021).

Neurobiology of Mood Disorders

Malfunctioning circuits across multiple brain regions and the underlying dysfunctional neurotransmission are implicated in the pathophysiology and the treatments for mood disorders. This has traditionally referred to neurocircuitry involving the monoamine neurotransmitters norepinephrine, dopamine, and serotonin. More recently, this perspective includes glutamate, gamma-aminobutyric acid (GABA), and their associated ion channels. Mood disorders are thought to involve dysfunction of various combinations of these neurotransmitters and ion channels. Thus, treatment options target these same neurotransmitters and ion channels. Understanding the receptors and pathways of these neurotransmitters, and how they interact to modulate the release of other neurotransmitters, forms a foundation for how they are involved in the pathophysiology and treatment of mood disorders.

Noradrenergic Pathways

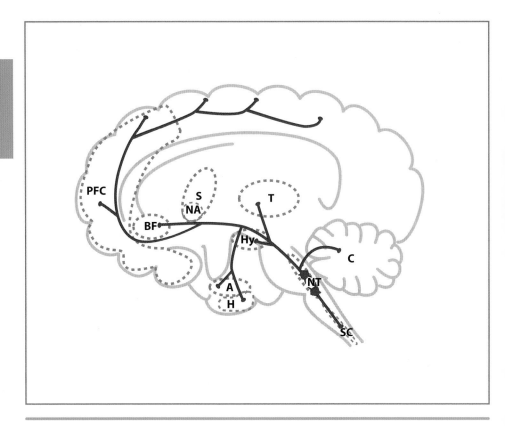

FIGURE 2.1. Norepinephrine has ascending and descending projections. The ascending pathways originate in the locus coeruleus of the brainstem and extend to multiple brain regions to regulate arousal, cognition, mood, and other functions. PFC, prefrontal cortex; BF, basal forebrain; S, striatum; NA, nucleus accumbens; T, thalamus; Hy, hypothalamus; A, amygdala; H, hippocampus; NT, brainstem neurotransmitter centers; SC, spinal cord; C, cerebellum (Stahl, 2021).

Norepinephrine Synthesis

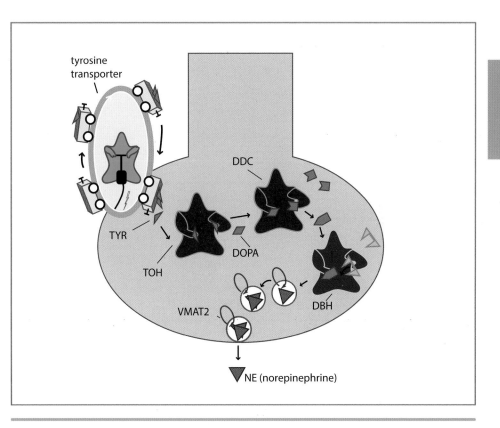

FIGURE 2.2. Norepinephrine is synthesized from the precursor amino acid, tyrosine, which is transported from the blood to the brain via an active transport pump. Inside the neuron, tyrosine is used to synthesize norepinephrine in a three-step sequential process: 1) the enzyme tyrosine hydroxylase (TOH) converts the amino acid tyrosine into DOPA. TOH is the most important and rate-limiting enzyme. 2) The enzyme DOPA decarboxylase (DDC) converts DOPA into dopamine (DA). 3) The enzyme dopamine β-hydroxylase (DBH) converts DA into norepinephrine (NE). After synthesis, NE is then packaged into vesicles via the vesicular monoamine transporter 2 (VMAT2) and stored until it is released into the synapse upon nerve conduction (Stahl, 2021).

Norepinephrine Action Is Terminated

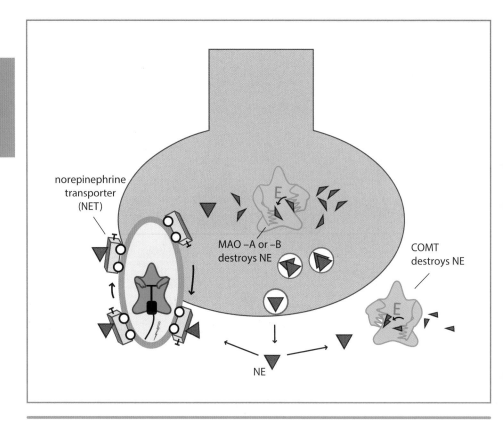

norepinephrine
transporter
(NET)

MAO –A or –B
destroys NE

COMT
destroys NE

NE

FIGURE 2.3. Norepinephrine can be terminated through a variety of mechanisms. NE can be transported out of the synaptic cleft and taken back into the presynaptic neuron via the norepinephrine transporter (NET), where it can be packaged for future use. Norepinephrine may alternatively be broken down intracellularly via monoamine oxidase A (MAO-A) and monoamine oxidase B (MAO-B), which are present in the mitochondria of the presynaptic neuron, and in other neurons and glia. Finally, NE may be broken down extracellularly via catechol-O-methyltransferase (COMT) (Stahl, 2021).

Norepinephrine Receptors

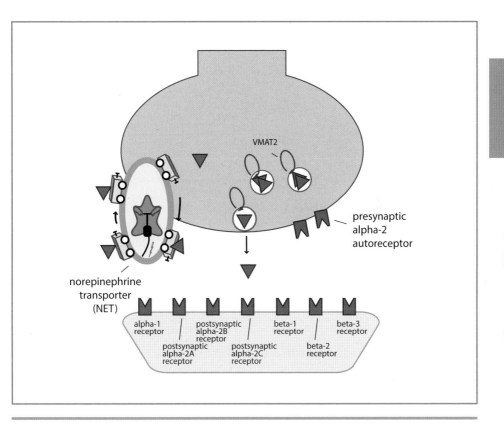

FIGURE 2.4. The receptors shown here regulate the transmission of norepinephrine. There is a presynaptic α2 autoreceptor, which regulates the release of norepinephrine from the presynaptic neuron. Both the terminal and somatodentritic α2 receptors are autoreceptors that act like a "brake" in a negative feedback system. When these receptors recognize NE, they stop the noradrenergic neuron from firing, thus regulating the amount of NE that gets released. Additionally, there are several postsynaptic receptors. These include α1, α2A, α2B, α2C, β1, β2, and β3 (Stahl, 2021).

Serotonergic Pathways

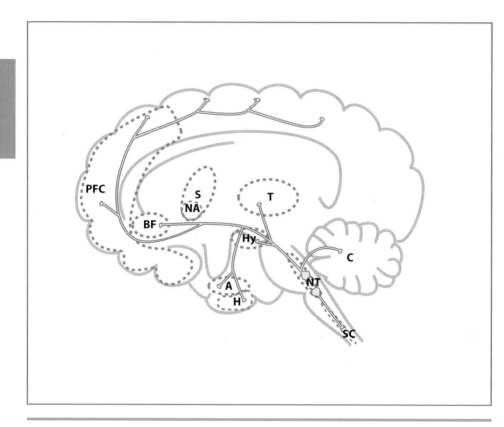

FIGURE 2.5. Like norepinephrine, serotonin has both ascending and descending projections. The ascending projections originate mostly in the raphe nucleus of the brainstem and project to many of the same regions as noradrenergic neurons. The ascending neurons regulate mood, sleep, anxiety, and additional functions. The descending pathways extend down the brainstem via the spinal cord and are thought to regulate pain. PFC, prefrontal cortex; BF, basal forebrain; S, striatum; NA, nucleus accumbens; T, thalamus; Hy, hypothalamus; A, amygdala; H, hippocampus; NT, brainstem neurotransmitter centers; SC, spinal cord; C, cerebellum (Stahl, 2021).

Serotonin Synthesis

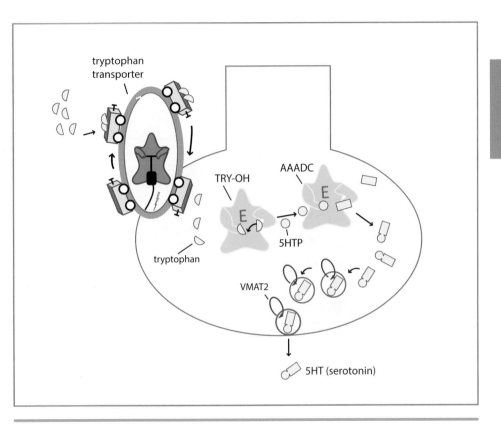

FIGURE 2.6. The synthesis of serotonin, also known as 5-hydroxytryptamine (5HT), begins after the amino acid precursor tryptophan is transported into the serotonin neuron. It is then converted by the enzyme tryptophan hydroxylase (TRY-OH) into 5-hydroxytryptophan (5HTP), which is then converted into 5HT by the enzyme aromatic amino acid decarboxylase (AAADC). Once synthesized, serotonin is then taken up into synaptic vesicles via the monoamine transporter (VMAT2), where it remains until released by neuronal impulse (Stahl, 2021).

Serotonin Action Is Terminated

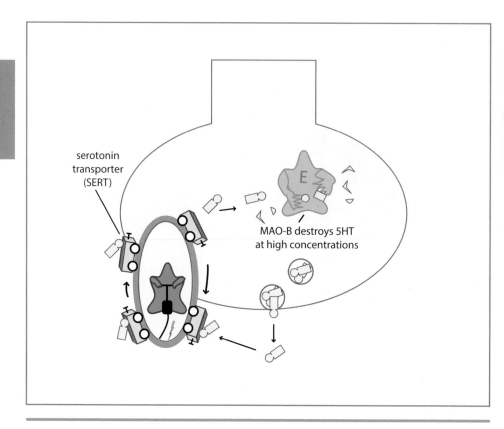

serotonin
transporter
(SERT)

MAO-B destroys 5HT
at high concentrations

FIGURE 2.7. Serotonin's action is terminated by the enzyme monoamine oxidase B (MAO-B) within the neuron when it is in high concentrations. This enzyme converts serotonin into an inactive metabolite. Excess serotonin is also cleared from the synapse and pulled back into the presynaptic neuron via the serotonin transporter (SERT), which is a presynaptic transport pump that is selective for serotonin (Stahl, 2021).

Serotonin Receptor Subtypes

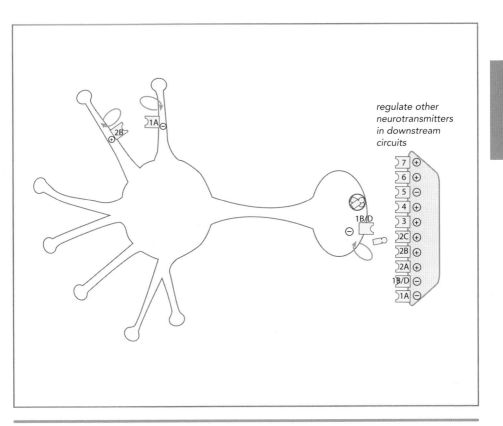

FIGURE 2.8. Serotonin has more than 12 receptors and at least half of them are known to have clinical significance. Only three receptors are located on the neuron itself: autoreceptors 5HT1A, 5HT1B/D, and 5HT2B. Presynaptically, these receptors monitor the firing, release, and storage of serotonin. These same receptors can also be located postsynaptically and have different functions there. Postsynaptically, there are also numerous serotonin receptors, which regulate other neurotransmitters in downstream circuits (Ohno et al., 2013; Stahl, 2021).

5HT Interacts in a Neuronal Network to Regulate All Major Neurotransmitter Systems

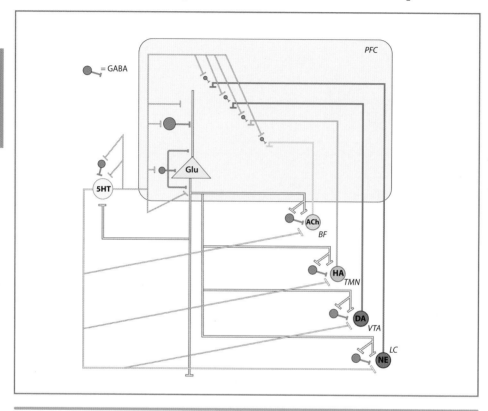

FIGURE 2.9. Serotonin circuits originate from discrete brainstem nuclei, including the dorsal and median raphe nuclei. These circuits project to a wide range of cortical and subcortical brain regions, including the prefrontal cortex (PFC). They also include loci for the cell bodies of neurons of other neurotransmitters, such as the locus coeruleus (LC) for norepinephrine, the ventral tegmental area (VTA) for dopamine, the tuberomammillary nucleus of the hypothalamus (TMN) for histamine (HA), and the basal forebrain (BF) for acetylcholine (ACh) (Mann, 2013; Stahl, 2021). The 5HT network may modulate itself directly and indirectly via these connections. These circuits influence virtually all other neurotransmitter networks. Therefore, it is not surprising that serotonin is thought to play a role in a variety of behaviors, such as mood, sleep, and appetite, and that disruption of serotonergic circuits has been implicated in many psychiatric disorders (Mann, 2013).

Dopaminergic Pathways

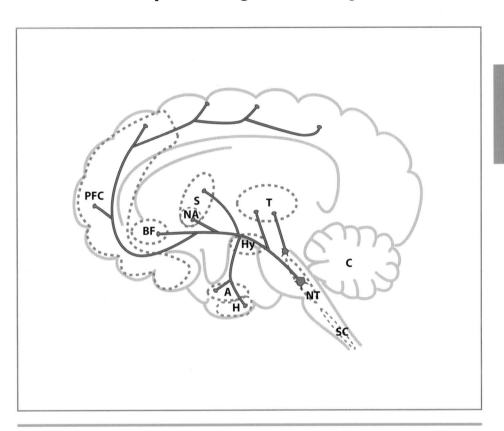

FIGURE 2.10. Dopamine has widespread ascending projections that originate predominantly in the brainstem (specifically the ventral tegmental area and the substantia nigra). These projections extend via the hypothalamus to the prefrontal cortex, basal forebrain, striatum, nucleus accumbens, and other regions. Dopaminergic neurotransmission is associated with cognition, pleasure and reward, movement, psychosis, and other functions. There are also direct projections from other sites to the thalamus, creating the "thalamic dopamine system." PFC, prefrontal cortex; BF, basal forebrain; S, striatum; NA, nucleus accumbens; T, thalamus; Hy, hypothalamus; A, amygdala; H, hippocampus; NT, brainstem neurotransmitter centers; SC, spinal cord; C, cerebellum (Stahl, 2021).

Dopamine Synthesis

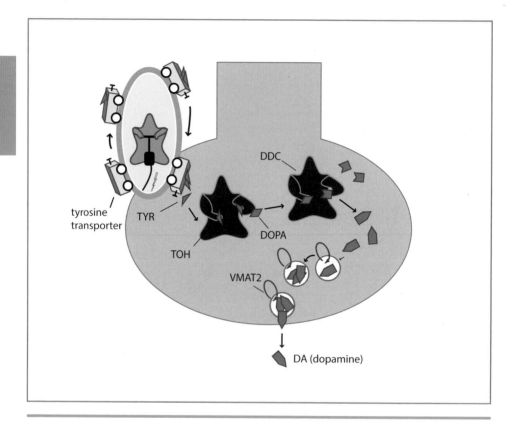

FIGURE 2.11. Dopamine synthesis begins when a precursor to dopamine, tyrosine (TYR), is taken up into dopamine nerve terminals via a tyrosine transporter. TYR is then converted into DOPA by the enzyme tyrosine hydroxylase (TOH). DOPA is then converted into dopamine by the enzyme DOPA decarboxylase (DDC). Once synthesized, dopamine is packaged into vesicles via the vesicular monoamine transporter (VMAT2) and stored there until its release into the synapse during neurotransmission (Stahl, 2021).

Dopamine Action Is Terminated

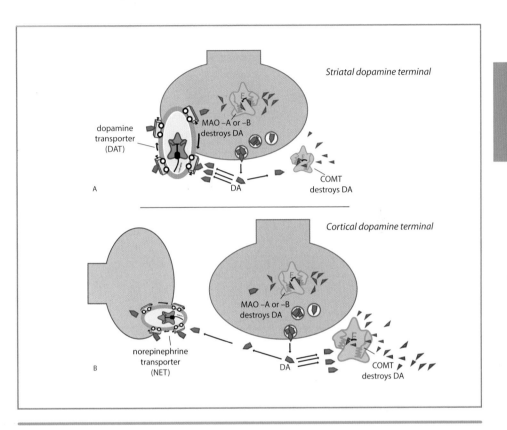

FIGURE 2.12. Dopamine's action is terminated through multiple mechanisms. A) Dopamine can be transported out of the synaptic cleft and pumped back into the presynaptic neuron via the dopamine transporter (DAT), where it can be repackaged for future use. Alternatively, dopamine may be broken down by monoamine oxidase A (MAO-A) and monoamine oxidase B (MAO-B), which are enzymes that are present in mitochondria inside the presynaptic neuron and other neurons and glia. Finally, dopamine may be broken down extracellularly via the enzyme catechol-O-methyltransferase (COMT). B) In the prefrontal cortex, DATs are scarce; thus, the predominant method of dopamine inactivation is via MAO-A or MAO-B intracellularly, or COMT extracellularly. Dopamine can also diffuse away from the synapse and be taken up by the norepinephrine transporter (NET) at neighboring neurons (Stahl, 2021).

Postsynaptic Dopamine Receptors

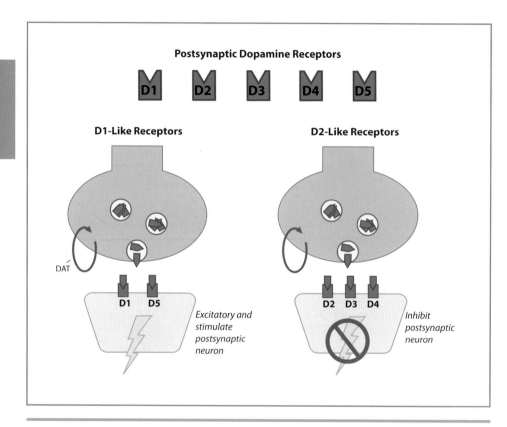

FIGURE 2.13. Dopamine receptors are the key regulators for dopaminergic neurotransmission. The DAT and VMAT2 are both types of receptors. There are many additional dopamine receptors, including at least five pharmacological subtypes, and several more molecular isoforms. Dopamine receptors are currently divided into two groups. The first group is the D1-like receptors including both D1 and D5 receptors. D1 receptors are excitatory and positively linked to adenylate cyclase. The second group is the D2-like receptors which includes D2, D3, and D4 receptors. These receptors are inhibitory and negatively associated with adenylate cyclase. Dopamine can be excitatory or inhibitory, depending on which dopamine receptor subtype it binds to. All five dopamine receptors can be located postsynaptically (Stahl, 2021).

Presynaptic Dopamine Receptors

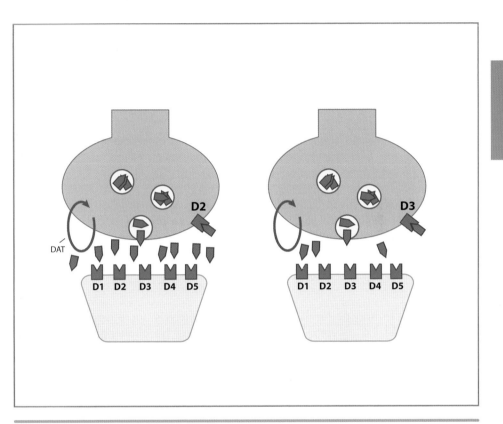

FIGURE 2.14. Dopamine 2 (D2) and dopamine 3 (D3) receptors are also located presynaptically, where they act as autoreceptors to inhibit further dopamine release. The D2 autoreceptor is less sensitive to dopamine than the D3 autoreceptor; thus, it takes a higher concentration of dopamine to activate the D2 autoreceptor compared to the D3 autoreceptor (Stahl, 2021).

Monoamine Receptor Actions Downstream

While we can to some extent associate changes in the synaptic amount of a particular neurotransmitter with clinical effects, in reality each neurotransmitter can bind to multiple receptors, with potentially divergent downstream effects at those different receptors (Ohno et al., 2013). What matters is in what brain region and at what receptors the neurotransmitters are binding to, not simply the level of the neurotransmitter.

The majority of the classic antidepressants are primarily serotonergic and work by blocking the 5HT transporter, effectively increasing levels of 5HT at the synapse throughout the brain and the body.

However, there are seven families of 5HT receptors with at least 14 subtypes, some that are presynaptic and directly influence the release of 5HT itself, and others that are postsynaptic and may influence the release of a myriad of different neurotransmitters (Ohno et al., 2013; Stahl, 2021). To complicate the situation further, some serotonin receptor subtypes are excitatory, while others are inhibitory.

When the 5HT transporter is blocked, this effectively increases 5HT, which can bind to all 14 receptor subtypes; thus, it can be challenging to predict exactly what the net effects linked to the therapeutic actions of a 5HT reuptake inhibitor may be. The results may be very individualized, depending on the unique receptor profile in a particular patient's brain. This profile might also be influenced by genetics, epigenetic processes, stress, psychotropic medications, or other factors. Understanding how 5HT receptors and receptor subtypes interact with each other to modulate the release of 5HT, as well as how they regulate the release of other neurotransmitters, is vital to understanding the mechanisms for potential therapeutic treatments for depression.

5HT Receptors Regulate 5HT Release: 1A, 1B, 1D, and 7

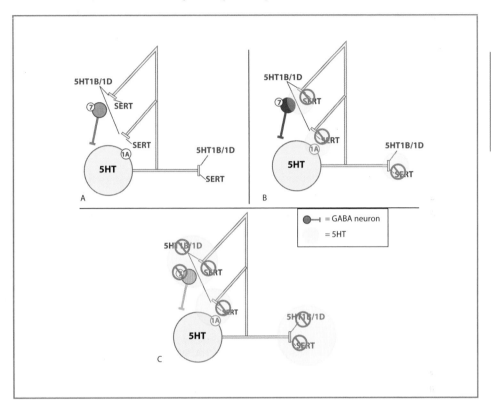

FIGURE 2.15. A) 5HT mostly regulates synaptic serotonin levels via the 5HT transporter, clearing excess 5HT from the synapse, but it also incorporates the use of presynaptic 5HT1A somatodendritic autoreceptors (Fink and Gothert, 2007) to regulate the amount of 5HT released. When 5HT binds to these receptors, it results in a shutdown of 5HT neuronal impulse and a decrease in 5HT released from the neuron terminal. Similarly, when 5HT binds to the 5HT1B and 1D receptors, found on the axon terminals, they shut down further release of 5HT. Finally, 5HT7 receptors that innervate GABA neurons in the raphe nucleus when activated stimulate the release of inhibitory GABA, which then turns off further 5HT release (Harshing et al., 2004; Sarkisyan et al., 2010). B) Blocking 5HT reuptake stimulates the 5HT autoreceptors to shut down 5HT release, which may explain the delayed therapeutic effects of 5HT reuptake inhibitors. C) Adding blockade or partial blockade of presynaptic 5HT1B and 1D receptors and postsynaptic 5HT7 receptors with simultaneous reuptake inhibition may enhance 5HT release.

5HT Receptors Regulate Glutamate Release Both Directly and Indirectly Part 1

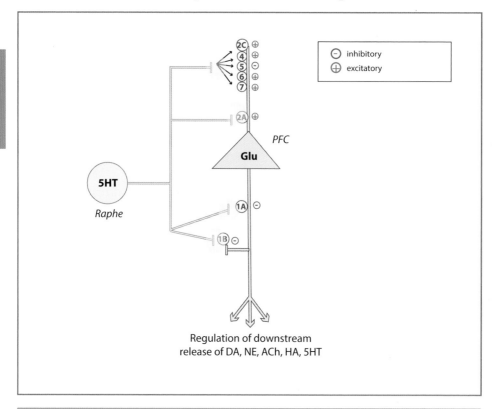

FIGURE 2.16A. Most 5HT receptor subtypes are postsynaptic heteroreceptors and exist on neurons that release any potential number of neurotransmitters. Thus, serotonin (like all neurotransmitters) can regulate downstream release of numerous neurotransmitters. 5HT's direct influence on glutamate pyramidal neurons can be both excitatory (e.g., at 5HT2A, 5HT2C, 5HT4, 5HT6, and 5HT7 receptors) and inhibitory (at 5HT1A, 5HT5, and potentially postsynaptic 5HT1B receptors). Glutamate neurons, effectively, synapse with the neurons of most other neurotransmitters to regulate their downstream release (Stahl, 2021).

5HT Receptors Regulate Glutamate Release Both Directly and Indirectly Part 2

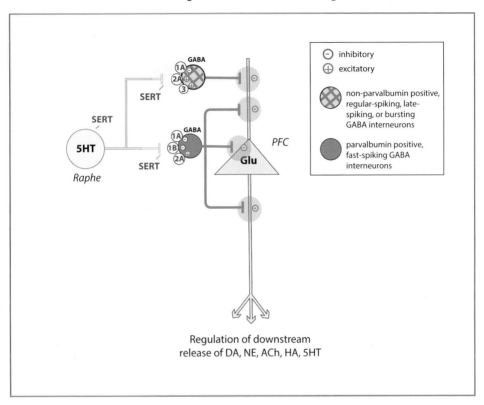

FIGURE 2.16B. Glutamate release can also be modulated indirectly by 5HT receptors on inhibitory GABAergic interneurons. With multiple ways to stimulate and inhibit glutamate neurons, and with some 5HT receptors having opposing actions on glutamate release due to their presence on both glutamate neurons and GABA interneurons (e.g., 5HT2A), it appears that the coordinated actions of 5HT at its various receptors may work to "tune" glutamate output and maintain balance (Kubota, 2014; Puig et al., 2010; Stahl, 2015a; Stahl, 2021). The net effects of 5HT upon glutamate release depend on the local concentration of 5HT, the regional and cellular expression patterns of 5HT receptor subtypes, and the density of the receptors.

5HT2A Receptors Regulate Glutamate Release — But It's Complicated

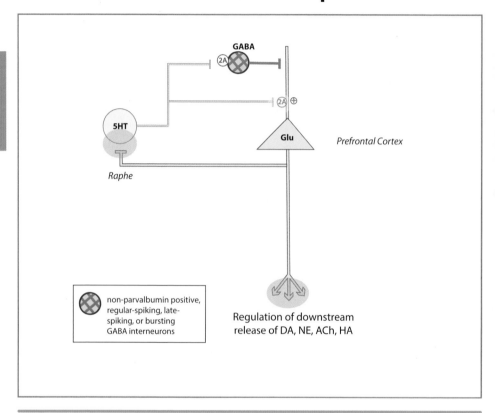

FIGURE 2.17A. The 5HT2A receptors are always excitatory; however, they can either stimulate or inhibit glutamate release, depending on their location (Artigas, 2013). 5HT2A receptors are located on glutamate pyramidal neurons and, through stimulation of these receptors, can increase glutamate release (Stahl, 2021).

5HT2A Receptors Regulate Glutamate Release—But It's Complicated

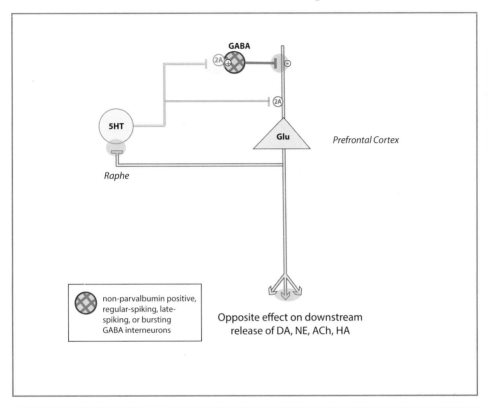

FIGURE 2.17B. 5HT2A receptors are also present on GABA interneurons and when stimulated cause inhibition of glutamate. Thus, the net effects of 5HT2A stimulation—or 5HT2A antagonism—on glutamate neurotransmission depends on multiple factors, including the local concentration of 5HT and the density of receptors (Artigas, 2013; Stahl, 2021).

Serotonin at 5HT3 Receptors Regulates Glutamate Release and Downstream Neurotransmitters

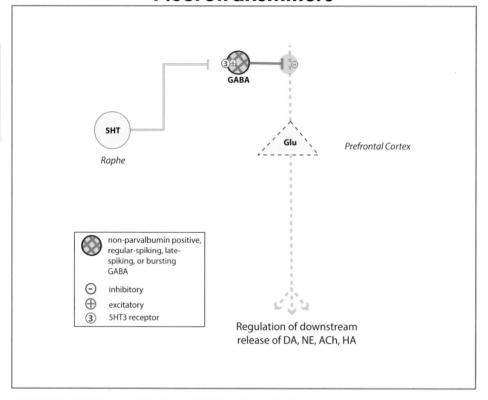

FIGURE 2.18A. Serotonin binding at 5HT3 receptors on GABA interneurons is excitatory; thus, it increases GABA. As a result, GABA inhibits glutamate pyramidal neurons, decreasing glutamate release. Reduced release of glutamate may lead to decreased release of downstream neurotransmitters, since pyramidal neurons synapse with neurons of most neurotransmitters (Stahl, 2021).

5HT3 Antagonists Disinhibit Glutamate Release and Enhance the Release of Downstream Neurotransmitters

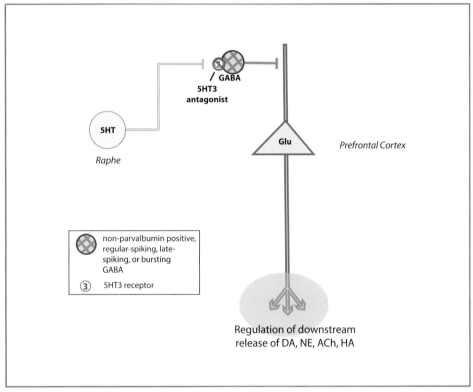

FIGURE 2.18B. Blocking the 5HT3 receptor removes GABA inhibition and disinhibits the pyramidal neurons. This increase in glutamate may result in the increased release of neurotransmitters downstream (Stahl, 2021).

5HT3 Receptors Regulate ACh and NE Release

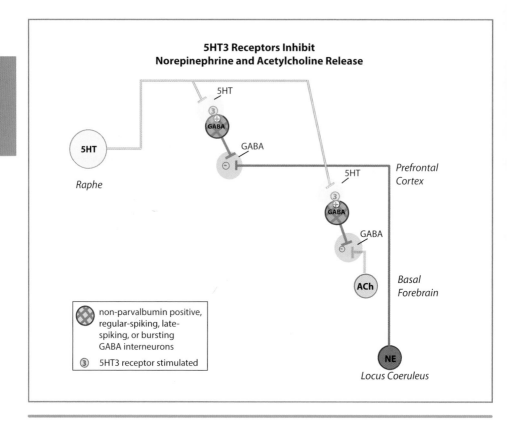

5HT3 Receptors Inhibit Norepinephrine and Acetylcholine Release

FIGURE 2.19. In the central nervous system (CNS), especially the prefrontal cortex, 5HT3 receptors are localized on a specific type of GABA interneuron with a characteristic firing pattern that is regular-spiking, late-spiking, or bursting (Artigas, 2013; Giovanni et al., 1998). 5HT3 receptors are excitatory upon the GABA neurons they innervate; thus, they have inhibitory effects. 5HT3 receptors specifically inhibit the release of acetylcholine (ACh) and norepinephrine (NE) at the cortical level. Interneurons with 5HT3 receptors terminate upon the nerve endings of presynaptic acetylcholine and norepinephrine neurons to inhibit them. Thus, 5HT3 antagonists, including some antidepressants, would be expected to have the opposite effect, resulting in increased levels of acetylcholine and norepinephrine (Artigas, 2013; Stahl, 2021).

5HT1A Heteroreceptors May Regulate the Release of Pro-Cognitive Neurotransmitters

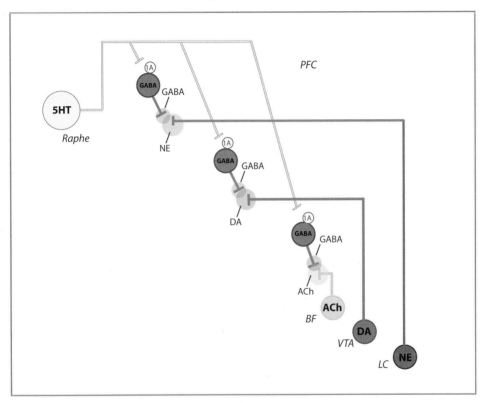

FIGURE 2.20. 5HT1A heteroreceptors on GABA interneurons in the prefrontal cortex can modulate the release of ACh, DA, and NE (Artigas, 2013; Carr and Lucki, 2011). Stimulation of 5HT1A receptors is inhibitory; thus, 5HT1A agonism or partial agonism could theoretically reduce GABA release and disinhibit ACh, DA, and NE release (Stahl, 2015b). The mechanism by which 5HT1A agonism modulates ACh, DA, and NE is still theoretical; however, if increased, these neurotransmitters are believed to have pro-cognitive effects.

Norepinephrine Modulates Other Neurotransmitters: Alpha-2 Receptors Part 1

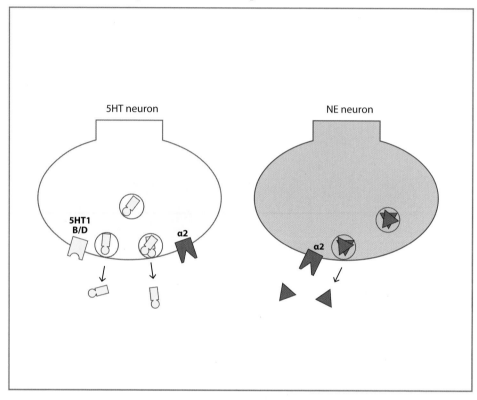

FIGURE 2.21A. Alpha-2 antagonism is another way to enhance the release of monoamines that has potential therapeutic effects in unipolar depression. On the left, a serotonergic neuron is shown with 5HT 1B/D autoreceptors and α2-adrenergic heteroreceptors. On the right, a noradrenergic neuron is shown with presynaptic α2 autoreceptors (Stahl, 2021).

Norepinephrine Modulates Other Neurotransmitters: Alpha-2 Receptors Part 2

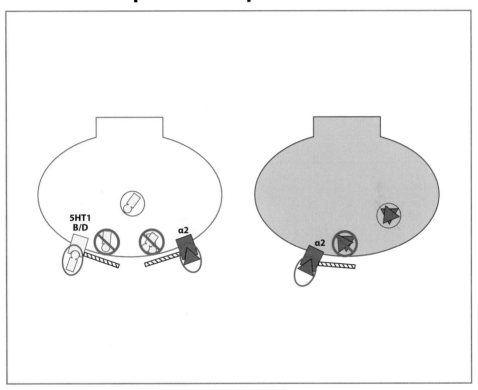

FIGURE 2.21B. On the left, both 5HT 1B/D autoreceptors and α2 heteroreceptors on serotonergic neurons function as "brakes" to terminate serotonin release when bound by their respective neurotransmitters. On the right, when norepinephrine binds to α2 autoreceptors on the norepinephrine neuron, this shuts off further norepinephrine release (Stahl, 2021).

Norepinephrine Modulates Other Neurotransmitters: Alpha-2 Receptors Part 3

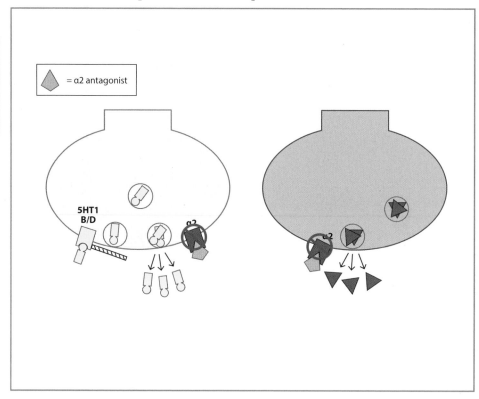

FIGURE 2.21C. Alpha-2 antagonists "cut the serotonin brake cable" when they block α2 presynaptic heteroreceptors, resulting in enhanced serotonin release (left). Alpha-2 antagonists also "cut the norepinephrine brake cable" by blocking presynaptic α2 autoreceptors, leading to enhanced norepinephrine release (right) (Stahl, 2021).

GABA Synthesis

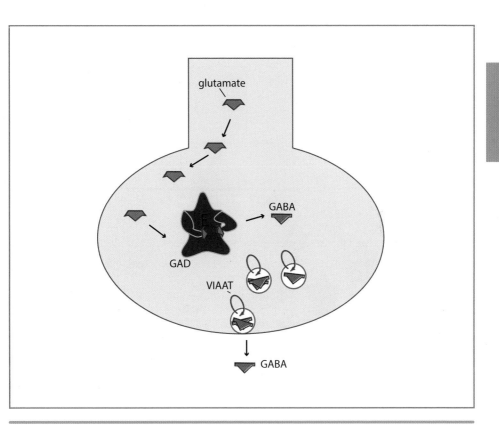

FIGURE 2.22. Glutamate, the precursor to GABA, is converted to GABA by the enzyme glutamic acid decarboxylase (GAD). Once synthesized, GABA is transported into synaptic vesicles via vesicular inhibitory amino acid transporters (VIAATs) and stored until its release into the synapse upon neurotransmission (Stahl, 2021).

GABA Action Is Terminated

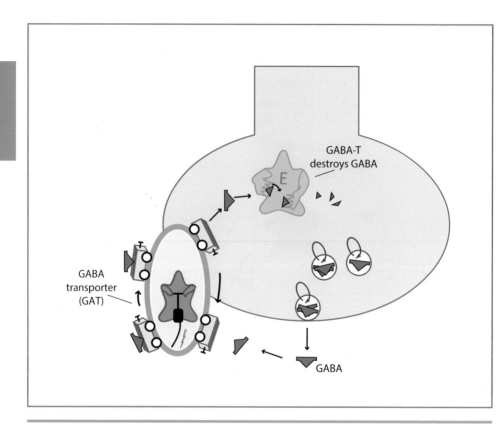

FIGURE 2.23. GABA's action can be terminated through a variety of mechanisms. GABA can be pumped back into the presynaptic neuron from the synaptic cleft by the GABA transporter (GAT), where it can be repackaged for future use. Once back in the presynaptic neuron, GABA may alternatively be converted into an inactive substance through the enzyme GABA transaminase (GABA-T) (Stahl, 2021).

GABA Receptors

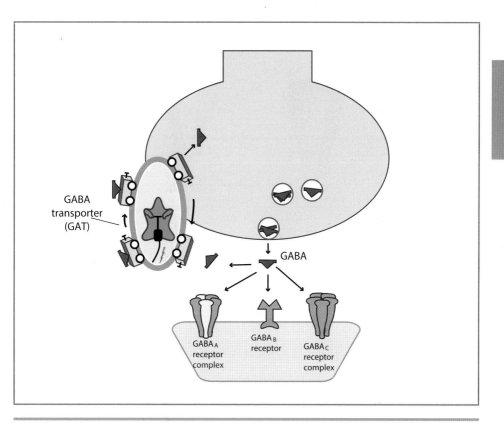

FIGURE 2.24. There are four major types of receptors that regulate GABA neurotransmission. The GABA transporter (GAT) is involved in pumping excess GABA from the synaptic cleft back into the presynaptic neuron. The three types of postsynaptic GABA receptors are: GABA$_A$, GABA$_B$, and GABA$_C$. GABA$_A$ and GABA$_C$ receptors are ligand-gated ion channels, meaning they are part of a macromolecular complex that forms a chloride ion channel. GABA$_B$ receptors are G-protein-linked receptors that may be coupled with potassium or chloride channels (Stahl, 2021).

Major Subtypes of GABA$_A$ Receptors

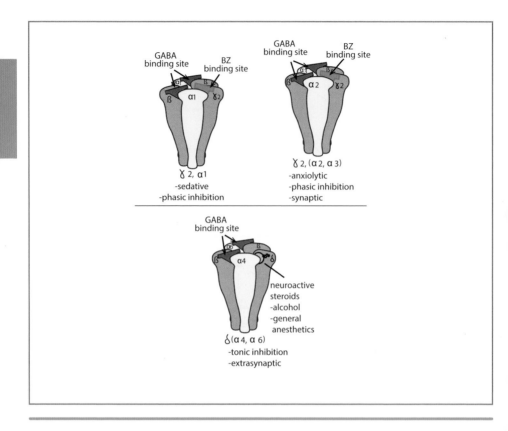

FIGURE 2.25. Four transmembrane proteins comprise one subunit of a GABA$_A$ receptor for a total of five subunits with a chloride channel in the middle. Different types of subunits (also called subunits and isoforms) can combine to form a GABA$_A$ receptor. The type and function of each GABA receptor will ultimately depend on which subunits it contains. Benzodiazepine-sensitive GABA$_A$ receptors (top two) contain two β units plus either a gamma-2 or gamma-3, plus two α (α1 through α3) subunits. They typically mediate phasic inhibition triggered by peak concentrations of synaptically released GABA. GABA$_A$ receptors containing the α4, α6, or delta subunits (bottom) are benzodiazepine-insensitive, are located extrasynaptically, and regulate tonic inhibition. They are activated by naturally occurring neuroactive steroids and potentially alcohol and some general anesthetics (Chen et al., 2019; Stahl, 2021).

Two Types of GABA$_A$-Mediated Inhibition

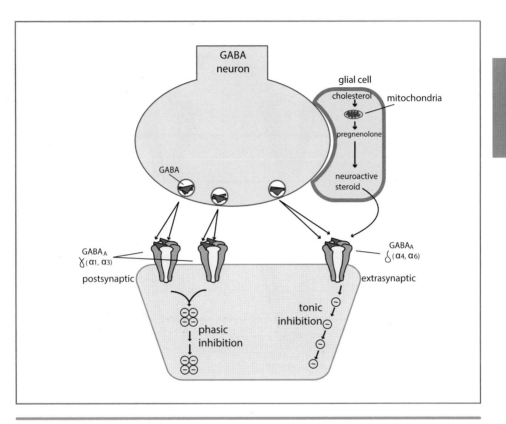

FIGURE 2.26. Benzodiazepine-sensitive GABA$_A$ receptors are postsynaptic receptors that mediate phasic inhibition, which occurs in bursts triggered by peak levels of synaptically released GABA. Benzodiazepine-insensitive GABA$_A$ receptors are extrasynaptic and capture GABA that diffuses away from the synapse, as well as neuroactive steroids that are produced and released by glia. They regulate tonic inhibition via ambient concentrations of extracellular GABA that has escaped from the synapse (Stahl, 2021).

Positive Allosteric Modulation of GABA$_A$ Receptors

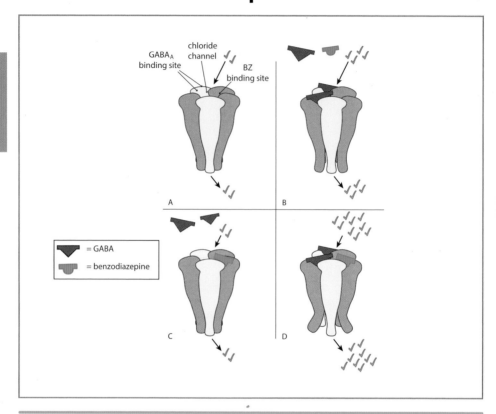

FIGURE 2.27. A) Benzodiazepine-sensitive GABA$_A$ receptors, like the one shown here, are comprised of five subunits with a central chloride channel and binding sites for GABA and positive allosteric modulators (e.g., benzodiazepines). B) When GABA binds to its sites on the GABA$_A$ receptor, it increases the frequency of opening of the chloride channel, allowing more chloride to pass through. C) When a positive allosteric modulator such as a benzodiazepine binds to the GABA$_A$ receptor in the absence of GABA, it has no effect on the chloride channel. D) When a benzodiazepine binds in the presence of GABA, it causes the channel to open more frequently than when GABA alone is present, thus modulating GABAergic neurotransmission (Alvarez et al., 2019; Stahl, 2021).

Glutamate Synthesis and Key Glutamate Pathways

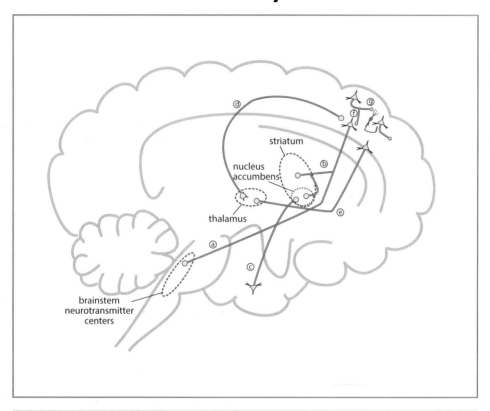

FIGURE 2.28. Glutamate, the major excitatory neurotransmitter, is theoretically hyperactive in some glutamate pathways in mania. It is also hypothesized to play a role in depression. Glutamate, or glutamic acid, is synthesized from glutamine in glia, cells that aid in the recycling and regeneration of additional glutamate following glutamate release in neurotransmission.

While glutamate can have actions at virtually all neurons, there are several major glutamatergic pathways. A) The cortico-brainstem glutamate pathway descends from the cortical pyramidal neurons in the prefrontal cortex (PFC) to the brainstem and regulates neurotransmitter release. B) Another pathway descends from the PFC to the striatal complex (cortico-striatal glutamate pathway) and is part of the cortico-striatal-thalamic loop, thought to control a variety of functions including attention, emotion, and executive function. C) A glutamatergic pathway projects from the ventral hippocampus to the nucleus accumbens. D) Thalamocortical glutamate pathways ascend from the thalamus and innervate pyramidal neurons in the cortex. E) Corticothalamic glutamate pathways descend from the PFC to the thalamus. F) Intracortical pyramidal cortical neurons can communicate directly with each other via the neurotransmitter glutamate. G) Intracortical neurons can also communicate via GABAergic interneurons; these indirect cortico-cortical glutamate pathways are therefore inhibitory (Stahl, 2021).

Glutamate Is Recycled and Regenerated
Part 1

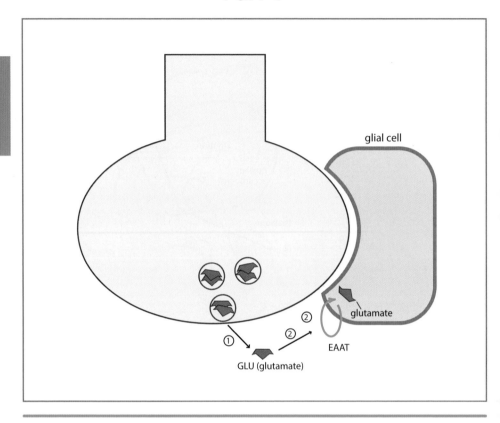

FIGURE 2.29A. After (1) release of glutamate from the presynaptic neuron, (2) it is taken up into glial cells via the excitatory amino acid transporter (EAAT).

Glutamate Is Recycled and Regenerated Part 2

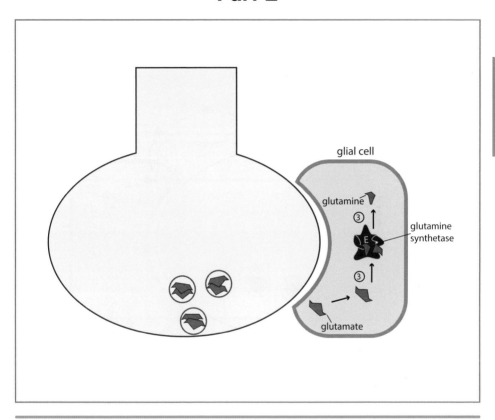

FIGURE 2.29B. Once inside the glial cell, glutamate is converted into glutamine by the enzyme glutamine synthetase (3).

Glutamate Is Recycled and Regenerated
Part 3

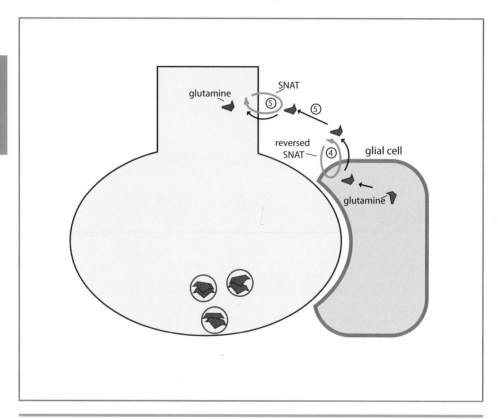

FIGURE 2.30A. Glutamine is released from glial cells by a specific glial neutral amino acid transporter (SNAT) through the process of reverse transport (4), and then taken up by SNATs on glutamate neurons (5).

Glutamate Is Recycled and Regenerated Part 4

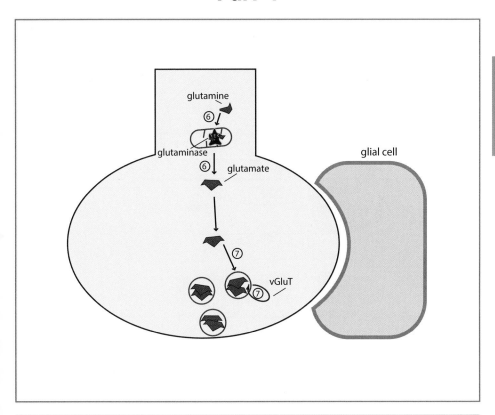

FIGURE 2.30B. Finally, glutamine is converted into glutamate within the presynaptic neuron by the enzyme glutaminase (6) and packaged into synaptic vesicles by the vesicular glutamate transporter (vGluT) (7), where it is stored for future release.

Glutamate Receptors

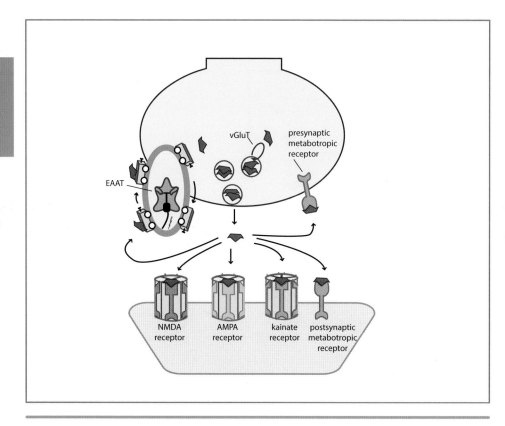

FIGURE 2.31. There are several types of glutamate receptors. The excitatory amino acid transporter (EAAT) is located on the presynaptic neuron and is responsible for clearing excess glutamate out of the synapse. The vesicular transporter (vGluT) transports glutamate into synaptic vesicles, where it is stored for future neurotransmission. Metabotropic receptors can occur presynaptically or postsynaptically. There are at least eight subtypes of metabotropic glutamate receptors, organized into three separate groups. Group II and III receptors can occur presynaptically where they function as autoreceptors to block glutamate release. Group I receptors are located primarily postsynaptically where they interact with other glutamate receptors to strengthen responses mediated by ligand-gated ion channel receptors. Three types of postsynaptic glutamate receptors are linked to ion channels and are known as ligand-gated ion channels: N-methyl-D-aspartate (NMDA) receptors, α-amino-3-hydroxy-5-methyl-4-isoxazole-propionic acid (AMPA) receptors, and kainate receptors, all named for the agonists that bind to them (Stahl, 2021).

From Circuits to Symptoms to Mechanisms of Treatments for Mood Disorders

Currently, a major hypothesis in psychiatry is that psychiatric symptoms are linked to inefficient information processing in specific brain circuits. Various circuits are thought to mediate different symptoms according to an evolving understanding of the distribution of functions across a variety of brain connections that form networks. To simplify, we may be able to associate specific nodes in the network with specific psychiatric symptoms.

The goal of this approach is to have a strategy for relieving all symptoms, in order to achieve complete remission, and to do so as rationally as possible based upon how those specific circuits are currently thought to be regulated by neurotransmitters in normal functioning and in psychiatric disorders. This strategy also involves rational use of the available medications that are known to target the regulation of those same neurotransmitters, and therefore to target improvement in the symptoms those neurotransmitters regulate.

Elucidating the relationship between symptoms of mood disorders, how they are connected to malfunctioning circuits in the brain, and how the underlying mechanisms may be used as targets for therapeutic treatment is essential to developing the most effective treatment strategies for individual patients.

Matching Mania Symptoms to Circuits

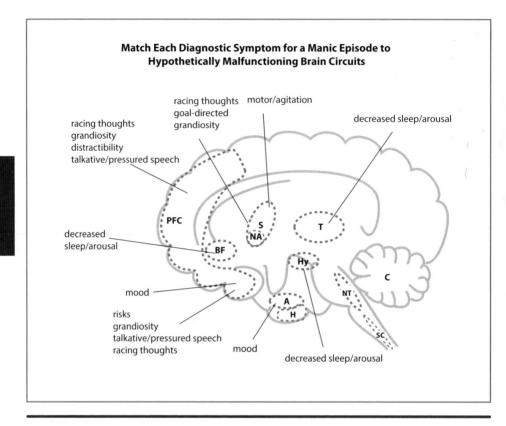

Match Each Diagnostic Symptom for a Manic Episode to
Hypothetically Malfunctioning Brain Circuits

FIGURE 3.1. Alterations in neurotransmission within each of the brain regions depicted here can be hypothetically linked to the various symptoms of a manic episode. Functionality in each brain region may be associated with a different constellation of symptoms. PFC, prefrontal cortex; BF, basal forebrain; S, striatum; NA, nucleus accumbens; T, thalamus; Hy, hypothalamus; A, amygdala; H, hippocampus; NT, brainstem neurotransmitter centers; SC, spinal cord; C, cerebellum (Stahl, 2021).

Matching Depression Symptoms to Circuits

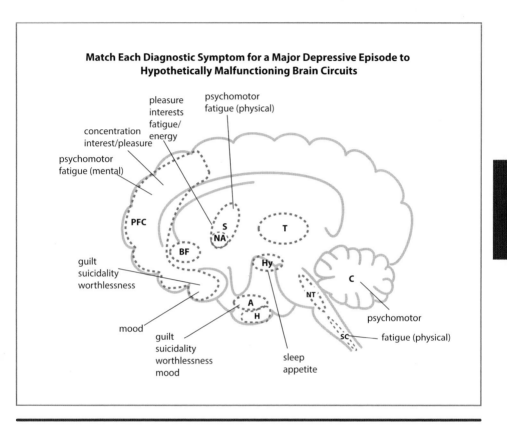

Match Each Diagnostic Symptom for a Major Depressive Episode to Hypothetically Malfunctioning Brain Circuits

FIGURE 3.2. Each of the nine symptoms listed for the diagnosis of a major depressive episode can be mapped onto brain circuits whose inefficient information processing theoretically controls these symptoms. Note the innervation of these various brain areas by the three monoamine neurotransmitter systems. Glutamate and GABA are ubiquitous throughout essentially every brain region. Each node in the networks that regulate psychiatric symptoms has neurotransmitters distributed to it in a unique if partially overlapping pattern that regulates each specific hypothetically malfunctioning brain circuit. Alterations in neuronal activity and in the efficiency of information processing within each of the brain regions shown here can lead to depressive symptoms. Targeting the relevant neurotransmitters that regulate those brain regions potentially results in reduction of each individual symptom. PFC, prefrontal cortex; BF, basal forebrain; S, striatum; NA, nucleus accumbens; T, thalamus; Hy, hypothalamus; A, amygdala; H, hippocampus; NT, brainstem neurotransmitter centers; SC, spinal cord; C, cerebellum (Stahl, 2021).

Circuits and Symptoms of Depression Part 1

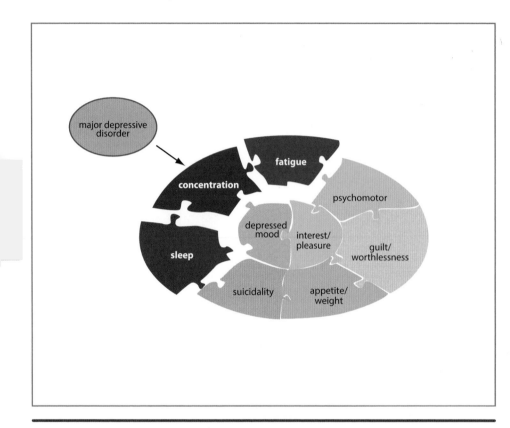

FIGURE 3.3. Shown here is the diagnosis of major depressive disorder deconstructed into its symptoms (as defined by the DSM-5-TR). Of these, concentration problems, fatigue, and sleep disturbances are the most common residual symptoms (Stahl, 2021).

Circuits and Symptoms of Depression Part 2

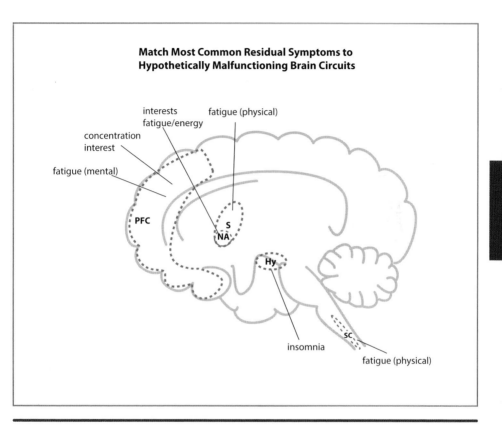

Match Most Common Residual Symptoms to Hypothetically Malfunctioning Brain Circuits

interests
fatigue/energy
concentration
interest
fatigue (mental)
fatigue (physical)

PFC

S
NA

Hy

SC
insomnia
fatigue (physical)

FIGURE 3.4. The most common residual symptoms of depression are linked to hypothetically malfunctioning brain circuits. Insomnia may be linked to the hypothalamus (Hy), concentration problems may be linked to the dorsolateral prefrontal cortex (DLPFC), reduced interest may be linked to the PFC and nucleus accumbens (NA), and fatigue may be linked to the PFC, striatum (S), NA, and spinal cord (SC). (Stahl, 2021).

Circuits and Symptoms of Depression Part 3

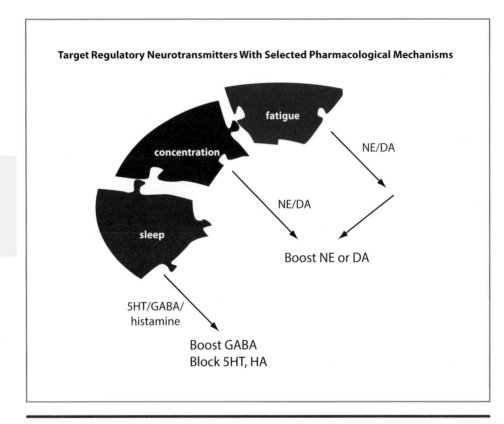

Target Regulatory Neurotransmitters With Selected Pharmacological Mechanisms

fatigue

concentration

sleep

NE/DA

NE/DA

5HT/GABA/
histamine

Boost NE or DA

Boost GABA
Block 5HT, HA

FIGURE 3.5. Residual symptoms of depression can be linked to the neurotransmitters that regulate them and then, in turn, to pharmacological mechanisms. Fatigue and concentration are regulated largely by norepinephrine (NE) and dopamine (DA) and thus may be treated by agents that increase NE and/or DA. Sleep disturbance is regulated by serotonin (5HT), gamma-aminobutyric acid (GABA), and histamine (HA), and thus could be treated with agents that boost GABA or block 5HT or HA (Stahl, 2021).

Response in Depression

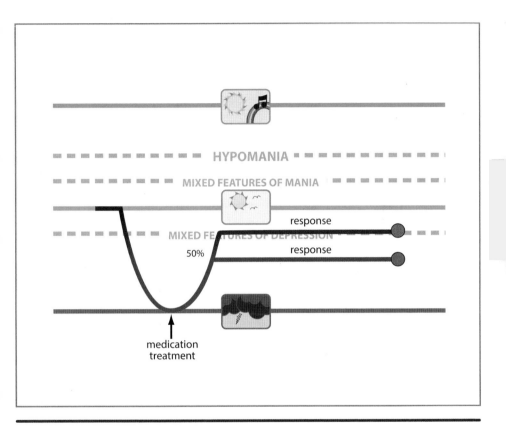

FIGURE 3.6. For patients with unipolar, bipolar, or mixed depression, who experience a major depressive episode, receive treatment, and improve to the level of 50% improvement in reduction of symptoms, it is called a response. Such patients are better but not completely well. Previously, this was considered the goal of depression treatment (Stahl, 2021).

Remission in Depression

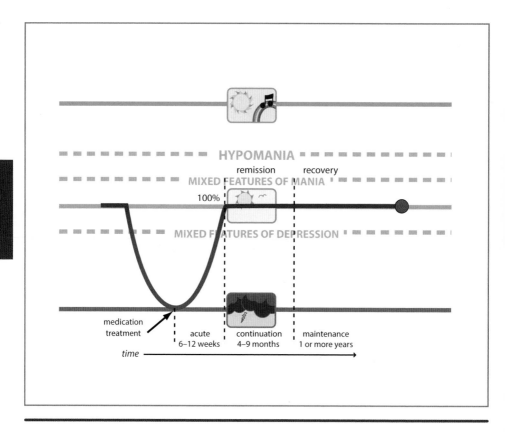

FIGURE 3.7. When treatment of a major depressive episode results in removal of essentially all symptoms, the patient is said to be in remission for the first few months. If this is sustained for longer than several months, it is referred to as recovery. Such patients are not just better, they are considered well. Remission and recovery are currently the goals when treating patients for depression (Stahl, 2021).

Relapse and Recurrence in Depression

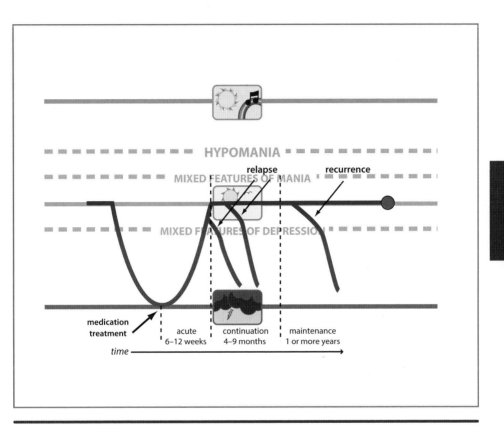

FIGURE 3.8. When depression returns before there is full remission of symptoms, or within the first several months following remission of symptoms, it is called relapse. When depression returns after a patient has recovered, it is called a recurrence (Stahl, 2021).

Remission in Depression

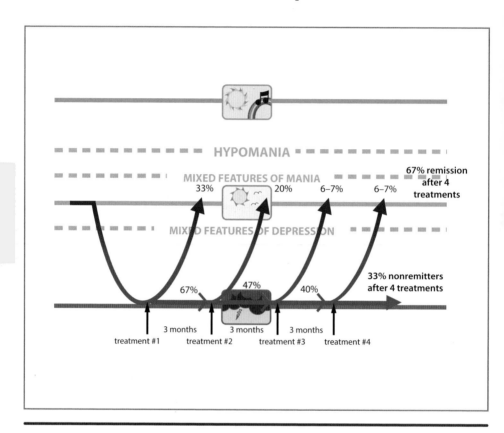

FIGURE 3.9. Approximately one-third of patients with unipolar depression will remit during any initial treatment (Little, 2009; Saveanu, 2015). Unfortunately, for those who fail to remit, the likelihood of remission with another monotherapy decreases with each successive trial. Thus, after a year of treatment with four sequential monotherapies taken for 12 weeks each, only two-thirds of patients will have achieved remission (Rush et al., 2006).

The rate of relapse of major depression is significantly less for patients who achieve remission. However, there is still risk of relapse even in remitters and the potential increases with the number of treatments it takes to get the patient to remit. Thus, relapse rates for patients who do not remit range from 60% at 12 months after one treatment to 70% at 6 months after four treatments (Rush et al., 2006). For those who do remit, the relapse rate ranges from only 33% at 12 months after one treatment all the way to 70% at 6 months after four treatments (Rush et al., 2006). In summary, the protective nature of remission virtually disappears once it takes four treatments to achieve remission (Grady and Stahl, 2015; Stahl, 2021).

Antidepressant Drugs for Unipolar Depression

The monoamines have traditionally played a major role in the therapeutic targets for the treatment of mood disorders; however, as the field advances, a variety of pharmacological mechanisms beyond monoamine reuptake have been discovered to be efficacious in the treatment of unipolar depression. We begin this section of the book with a focus on selective serotonin reuptake inhibitors (SSRIs) with unique pharmacological properties. We also include serotonin-norepinephrine reuptake inhibitors (SNRIs), norepinephrine-dopamine reuptake inhibitors (NDRIs), and serotonin partial agonist reuptake inhibitors (SPARIs) that are evidence-based for the treatment of unipolar depression. Finally, we explore drugs with mechanisms beyond monoamine reuptake and examine their unique properties.

Selective Serotonin Reuptake Inhibitors (SSRIs)

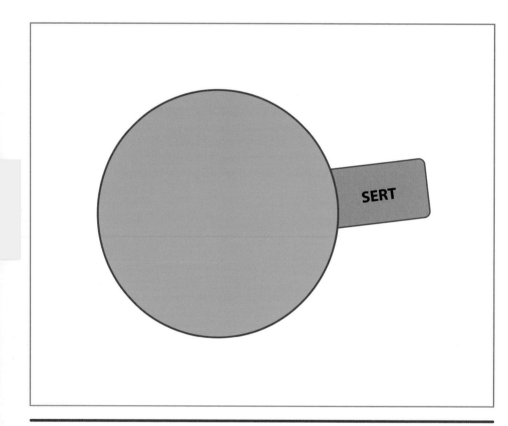

FIGURE 3.10. Selective serotonin reuptake inhibitors (SSRIs) transformed the field of clinical psychopharmacology. Some estimate that SSRI prescriptions in the United States (US) alone occur at the rate of seven prescriptions per second, estimating over 225 million a year (Stahl, 2021). Clinical indications for use of SSRIs range far beyond unipolar major depressive disorder. There are six principal agents in this group that we will address in this book. Each of these drugs belong to the SSRI class of drugs; however, they each have additional unique pharmacological properties that allow them to be distinguished from one another.

SSRI Action

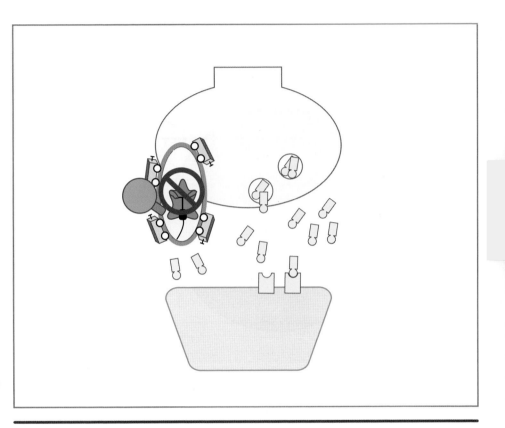

FIGURE 3.11. The serotonin reuptake inhibitor utilizes a mechanism described in its name to block the serotonin transporter or SERT, thus increasing the availability of serotonin in the synapse. According to the monoamine hypothesis, there is a relative deficiency in serotonin (5HT). According to the neurotransmitter receptor hypothesis of depression, both presynaptic 5HT1A autoreceptors and postsynaptic 5HT receptors are upregulated. When an SSRI is administered, and the SERT is blocked, this causes an initial increase in 5HT only in the somatodendritic areas of the 5HT neuron. The increased serotonergic binding at the somatodendritic 5HT1A autoreceptors results in desensitization or downregulation of these receptors. Once this occurs, there is no longer inhibition of impulse flow in the neuron, resulting in increased release of 5HT from the axon terminals into the synapse. This increase of 5HT at the axon causes the postsynaptic receptors to desensitize/downregulate, reducing side effects (Stahl, 2021).

Fluoxetine

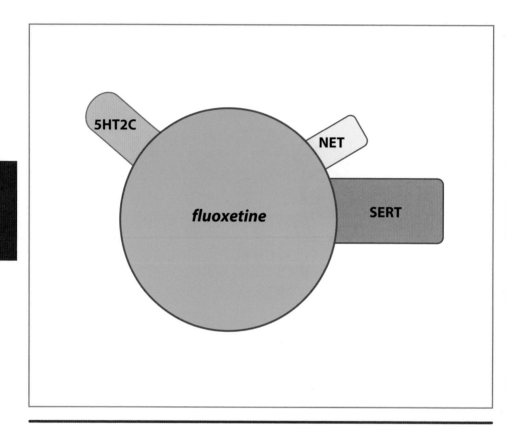

FIGURE 3.12. In addition to serotonin reuptake inhibition, fluoxetine has norepinephrine reuptake inhibition (NRI) and serotonin 2C antagonist actions (5HT2C). 5HT2C antagonism can lead to disinhibition of norepinephrine and dopamine. This action may be responsible for fluoxetine's activating effects. The NRI mechanism may be clinically relevant only at very high doses. Fluoxetine is not only available as a once-daily formulation, but also as a once-weekly oral dosage formulation (Stahl, 2021).

Sertraline

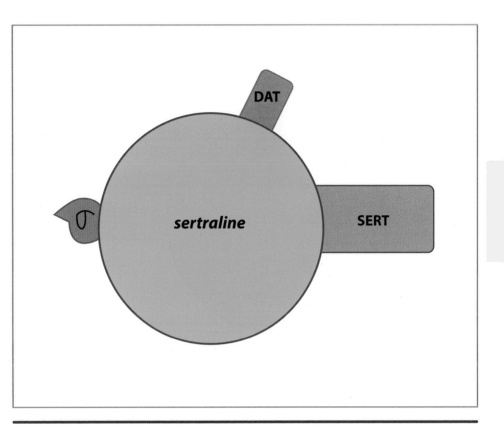

FIGURE 3.13. Sertraline has dopamine transporter inhibition and sigma-1 receptor binding in addition to serotonin reuptake inhibition (SRI). The clinical relevance of sertraline's DAT inhibition is unknown, although it may improve energy, concentration, and motivation. Its sigma properties may contribute to anxiolytic actions and may be helpful in patients with psychotic depression (Stahl, 2021).

Paroxetine

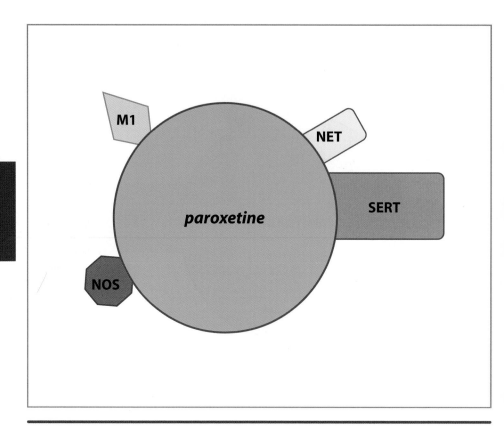

FIGURE 3.14. In addition to serotonin reuptake inhibition, paroxetine has mild anticholinergic actions (M1), which can be calming or potentially sedating, weak norepinephrine transporter (NET) inhibition, which may contribute to further antidepressant actions, and inhibition of the enzyme nitric oxide synthase (NOS), which may contribute to sexual dysfunction (Stahl, 2021).

Fluvoxamine

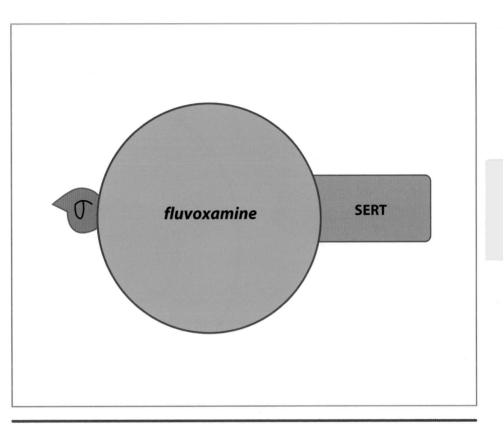

FIGURE 3.15. Fluvoxamine has serotonin reuptake inhibition action with additional properties. Like sertraline, fluvoxamine binds to sigma-1 sites; however, this action is more potent for fluvoxamine. The physiological function of the sigma-1 sites is still not completely understood; however, it has been linked to both anxiety and psychosis. Preclinical studies suggest that fluvoxamine may be an agonist at sigma-1 receptors, and that this property may contribute to its well-known anxiolytic properties (Stahl, 2021).

Citalopram

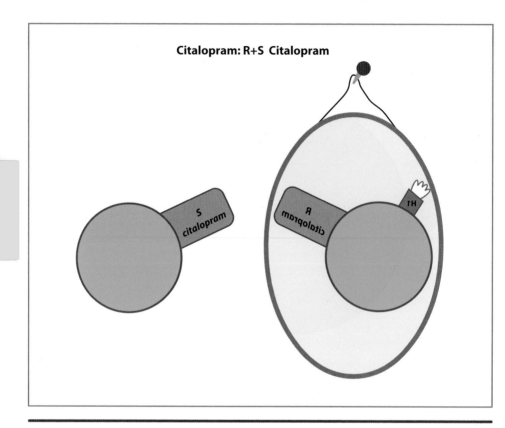

Citalopram: R+S Citalopram

FIGURE 3.16. Citalopram consists of two enantiomers, R and S, which are mirror images of each other. The mixture of these is known as racemic citalopram, but is commonly called citalopram. Some pharmacological evidence suggests that the R enantiomer may be pharmacologically active at SERTs in a manner that does not inhibit SERTs but actually interferes with the ability of the active S enantiomer to inhibit SERTs. The R enantiomer also has weak antihistamine properties. Racemic citalopram is generally one of the better-tolerated SSRIs and has favorable findings in the treatment of depression in elderly people, but has somewhat inconsistent therapeutic action at the lowest dose, often requiring dose increase to optimize treatment. However, this is challenging because dose increase is limited, due to the potential QTc prolongation at higher doses. All of these factors suggest that it is not favorable for citalopram to include the R enantiomer (Stahl, 2021).

Escitalopram

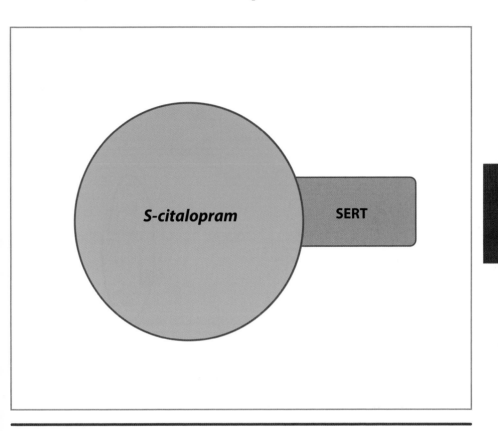

FIGURE 3.17. While the R and S enantiomers are mirror images of each other, they have slightly different clinical properties. Removing the R enantiomer with unwanted properties, and creating a drug that consisted of the pure S enantiomer, resulted in escitalopram. By removing the R enantiomer, this removes the antihistaminergic properties and there is no longer the high dose restriction to avoid QTc prolongation. Additionally, removing the potentially interfering R enantiomer makes the lowest dose of escitalopram efficacious. Thus, it is likely that pure SERT inhibition explains almost all of its pharmacological actions. Escitalopram is considered perhaps the best-tolerated SSRI, with the fewest cytochrome P450 (CYP450)-mediated drug interactions (Stahl, 2021).

Mechanisms of Serotonin Partial Agonist Reuptake Inhibitors

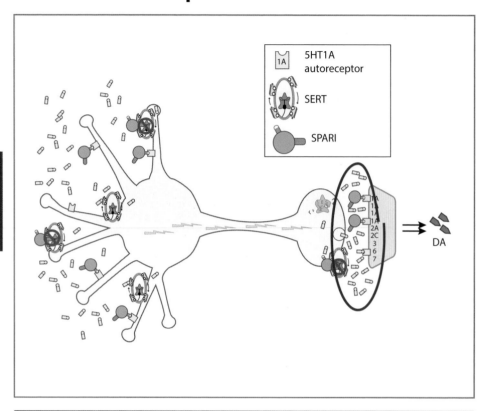

FIGURE 3.18. When a serotonin partial agonist reuptake inhibitor (SPARI) is administered, about half of serotonin transporter (SERTs) and half of serotonin 1A (5HT1A) receptors are occupied immediately. Blockade of the SERTs causes serotonin to increase initially in the somatodendritic area of the serotonin neuron. As a consequence of the increased SERTs, the somatodendritic 5HT1A autoreceptors desensitize or downregulate. When this occurs, there is no longer inhibition of impulse flow in the serotonin neuron, resulting in the neuronal impulse being turned on, and increasing the amount of 5HT released into the synapse by the axon terminal. Finally, there may be desensitization of the postsynaptic 5HT receptors (depicted in the figure by the absence of most postsynaptic receptors next to their receptor numbers). The addition of the 5HT1A partial agonism may lead to downstream enhancement of dopamine (DA) release, which may mitigate sexual dysfunction (Stahl, 2021).

Vilazodone

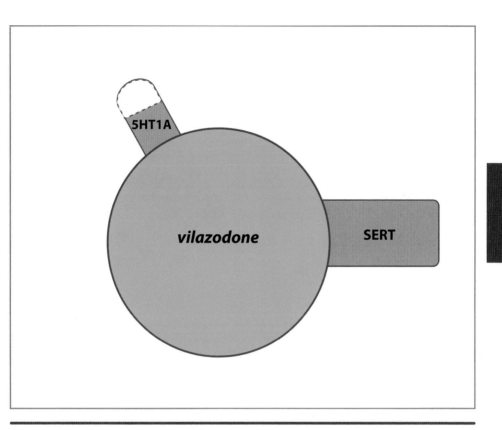

FIGURE 3.19. Vilazodone is a partial agonist at the serotonin 1A receptor and also inhibits serotonin reuptake. For these reasons, it is referred to as a serotonin partial agonist reuptake inhibitor (SPARI). 5HT1A immediate partial agonist actions are theoretically additive or synergistic with simultaneous SERT inhibition. Since this leads to faster and more robust actions at 5HT1A somatodendritic autoreceptors than with SERT inhibition alone, the mechanism results in faster and more robust elevation of synaptic 5HT (Schwartz et al., 2011; Stahl, 2014a; Stahl, 2021).

Mechanisms of Serotonin-Norepinephrine Reuptake Inhibitors (SNRIs)

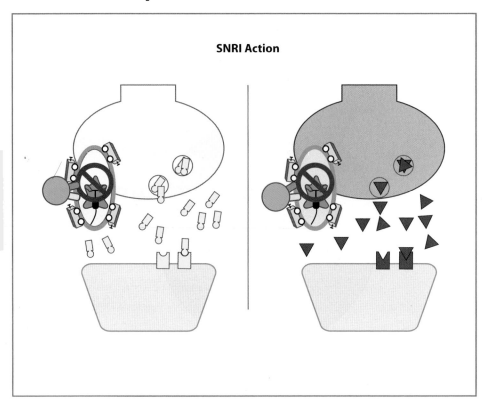

FIGURE 3.20. The mechanism underlying SNRIs has dual action. Both the serotonin reuptake inhibitor portion of the SNRI molecule (left panel) and the norepinephrine reuptake inhibitor portion of the SNRI molecule (right panel) are inserted into their respective reuptake pumps. Consequently, both pumps are blocked, and synaptic serotonin and norepinephrine are increased (Stahl, 2021).

Venlafaxine/Desvenlafaxine

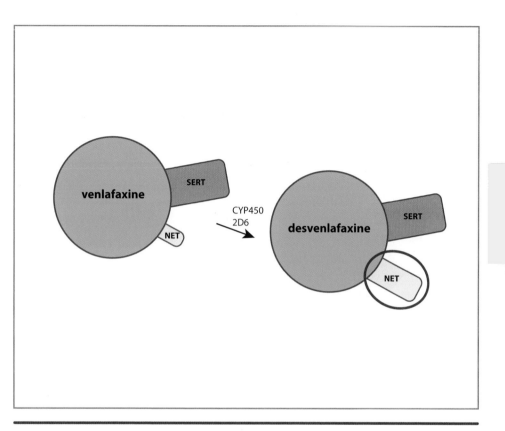

FIGURE 3.21. Venlafaxine inhibits both the serotonin transporter (SERT) and the norepinephrine transporter (NET), thus combining two therapeutic mechanisms in one agent. Venlafaxine's serotonergic actions are present at low doses, while its noradrenergic properties are progressively enhanced as the dose increases. Venlafaxine is converted to its active metabolite, desvenlafaxine, by CYP450 2D6. Like venlafaxine, desvenlafaxine inhibits reuptake of serotonin and norepinephrine; however, its NET actions are more potent relative to its SERT actions compared to venlafaxine. Venlafaxine administration usually results in plasma levels of venlafaxine that are about half those of desvenlafaxine. However, this can vary depending on genetic polymorphisms of CYP450 2D6 and if patients are taking medications that are inhibitors or inducers of CYP450 2D6 (Stahl, 2021).

Duloxetine

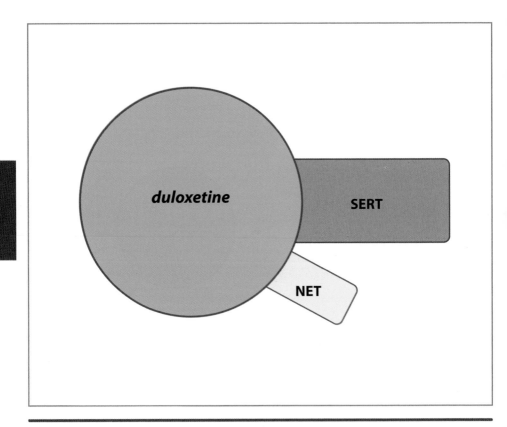

FIGURE 3.22. Duloxetine inhibits both the SERT and the NET (Stahl, 2021). Its noradrenergic actions may contribute to efficacy for painful physical symptoms. This SNRI, characterized by slightly stronger SERT than NET inhibition, has transformed the way that we view depression and pain. This SNRI relieves unipolar depression in the absence of pain, and it also relieves pain in the absence of depression. A variety of pain conditions are improved with this SNRI, from diabetic peripheral neuropathy, to fibromyalgia, to conditions associated with low back pain and more. Research on duloxetine has established efficacy not only in unipolar depression and in chronic pain, but also in patients with chronic painful physical symptoms of unipolar depression. Duloxetine has also shown to be efficacious in the treatment of cognitive symptoms of depression that are prominent in geriatric depression (Raskin et al., 2007).

S-milnacipran (levo)

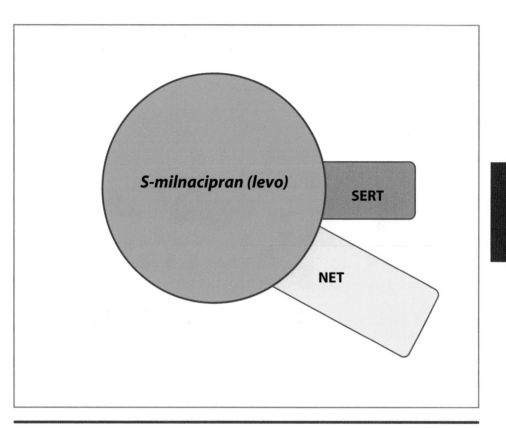

FIGURE 3.23. Milnacipran is a racemic mixture of two enantiomers. The racemic mixture is only approved for fibromyalgia and not unipolar depression in the United States (US). The S or levo enantiomer is the active enantiomer and has been independently developed for unipolar depression in the US, where it is mostly available. Like racemic milnacipran, levomilnacipran has greater NET inhibition than SERT inhibition and may target fatigue and lack of energy as potential clinical advantages. It is dosed in a controlled-release formulation, so unlike racemic milnacipran, it can only be given once a day. (Stahl, 2021).

Mechanisms of Norepinephrine-Dopamine Reuptake Inhibitors (NDRIs)

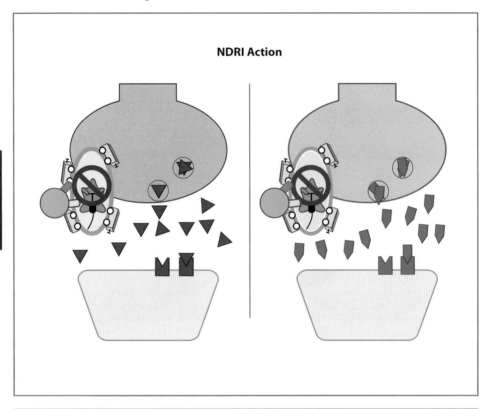

FIGURE 3.24. The norepinephrine reuptake inhibitor portion of the NDRI molecule (left panel) and the dopamine reuptake inhibitor portion of the NDRI molecule (right panel) are inserted into their respective reuptake pumps. With both pumps blocked, synaptic norepinephrine and dopamine are increased. NDRIs have unique effects in the prefrontal cortex. Since the prefrontal cortex lacks dopamine transporters (DATs) and NETs transport dopamine (DA) in addition to norepinephrine (NE), NET blockade also leads to an increase in synaptic DA in the prefrontal cortex. Thus, despite the absence of DATs in the prefrontal cortex, NDRIs still increase DA there. In contrast, the striatum has DATs and inhibition of these is responsible for the increase in DA there (Stahl, 2021).

Bupropion

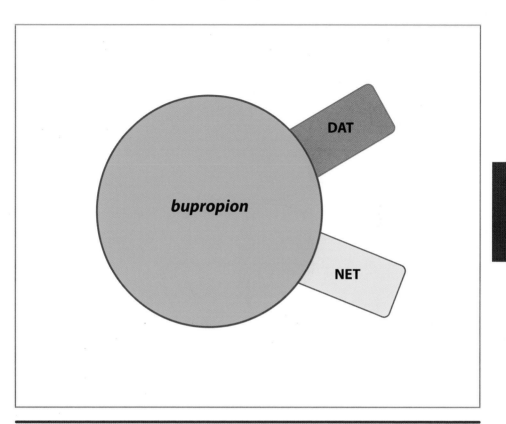

FIGURE 3.25. The prototypical norepinephrine-dopamine reuptake inhibitor (NDRI) is bupropion. Bupropion has weak blocking properties for the dopamine transporter (DAT) and for the norepinephrine transporter (NET). Its antidepressant actions may be explained in part by the more potent inhibitory properties of its metabolites (Stahl, 2021).

Beyond Monoamine Reuptake Inhibition: Serotonin Antagonist/Reuptake Inhibitors (SARIs) Part 1

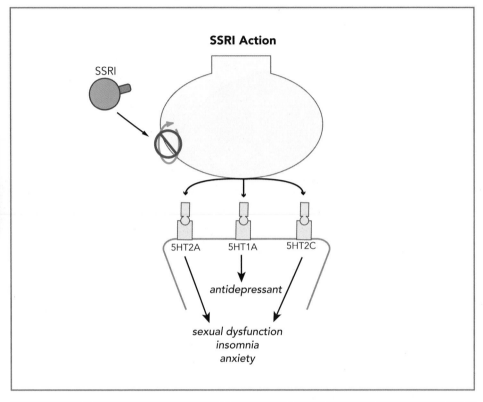

FIGURE 3.26A. There are several evidence-based treatments for unipolar depression with additional properties beyond monoamine reuptake inhibition. SSRIs block the serotonin transporter (SERT) at the presynaptic neuron, increasing serotonin at all receptors, with 5HT1A-mediated antidepressant actions, but also 5HT2A- and 5HT2C-mediated sexual dysfunction, insomnia, and anxiety (Stahl, 2021).

Beyond Monoamine Reuptake Inhibition: Serotonin Antagonist/Reuptake Inhibitors (SARIs) Part 2

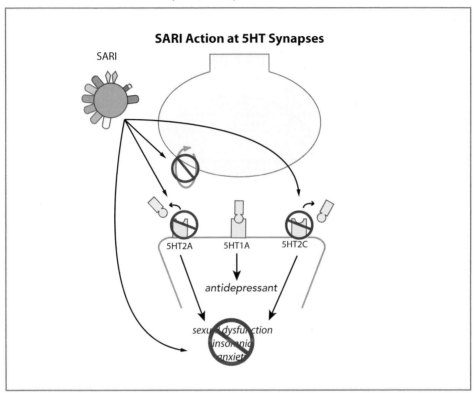

FIGURE 3.26B. One example of an agent with additional properties beyond reuptake is a drug that blocks serotonin 2A and 2C receptors and also functions as an SSRI. These are called serotonin antagonist/reuptake inhibitors (SARIs). SERT inhibition by a serotonin 2A antagonist/reuptake inhibitor at the presynaptic neuron increases serotonin at 5HT1A receptors, resulting in antidepressant actions. However, SARI action also blocks serotonin at 5HT2A and 5HT2C receptors, thus preventing sexual dysfunction, insomnia, or anxiety. Blocking these receptors can actually result in improved sleep, reduced anxiety, and decreased sexual dysfunction, potentially independently improving depressive symptoms (Stahl, 2021).

Trazodone

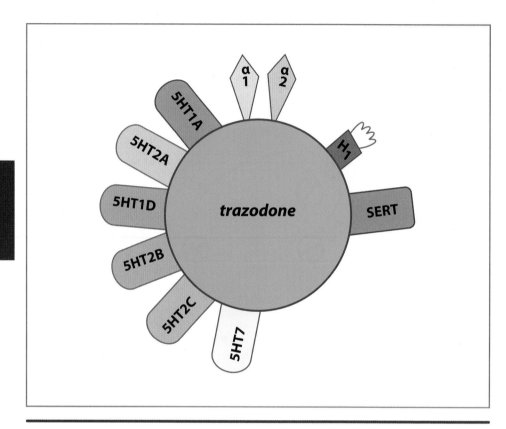

FIGURE 3.27. The prototype serotonin antagonist/reuptake inhibitor (SARI) is trazodone. It is a medication that blocks serotonin 2A and 2C in addition to serotonin reuptake. Trazodone acts very differently depending on the dose and the formulation. A more complete image of trazodone's binding properties has been elucidated, based on recent studies. It has antagonist actions at 5HT2A and 5HT2C receptors, but also at 5HT1D, 5HT2B, and 5HT7 receptors. In addition, trazodone has potent antagonist properties at α1B, α1A, α2C, and α2B receptors, H1 histamine receptors, and agonist actions at 5HT1A receptors. Because these various pharmacological actions occur with varying potencies, trazodone will act predominantly via its highest-affinity receptor interactions at low doses and will recruit its lower-affinity receptor actions at higher doses (Settimo and Taylor, 2018). High doses of 150–600mg that recruit the serotonin transporter (SERT) are required for trazodone to have therapeutic actions in depression. At lower doses it is an effective agent for treating insomnia. Trazodone extended release (XR) given once nightly at 300mg generates plasma levels that rise slowly and never fall below minimum antidepressant concentrations (Stahl, 2021).

Agomelatine

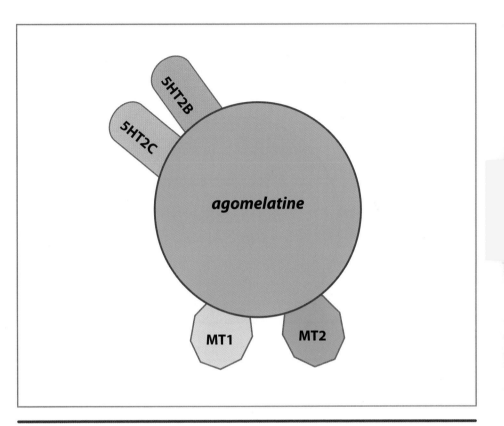

FIGURE 3.28. Agomelatine is approved to treat unipolar depression in many countries outside of the US. It has agonist actions at melatonin 1 (MT1) and melatonin 2 (MT2) receptors and antagonist actions at 5HT2C receptors. The 5HT2C antagonist actions are a property of several drugs used to treat unipolar depression. 5HT2C receptors are located in the midbrain raphe and prefrontal cortex (PFC) where they regulate the release of dopamine (DA) and norepinephrine (NE), which is believed to improve depressive symptoms (Stahl et al., 2010; Stahl, 2014b; Zajecka et al., 2010). Normally, serotonin binding at 5HT2C receptors on the gamma-aminobutyric acid (GABA) interneurons in the brainstem inhibits NE and DA release in the PFC. When a 5HT2C antagonist such as agomelatine binds to 5HT2C receptors on GABA interneurons it prevents serotonin (5HT) from binding there and therefore prevents inhibition of NE and DA release in the PFC. In other words, it disinhibits their release, resulting in increased levels. Agomelatine may also improve depressive symptoms by resynchronizing circadian rhythms, acting as a "substitute melatonin" (Stahl, 2021).

Mirtazapine

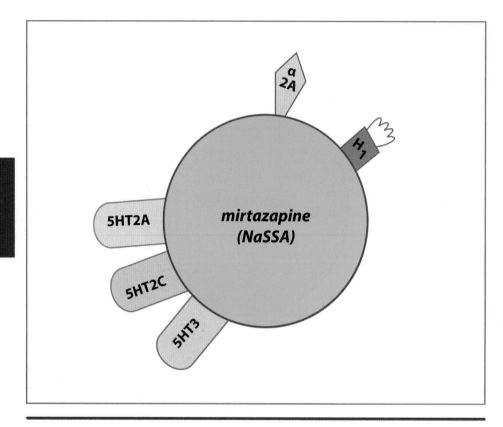

FIGURE 3.29. Mirtazapine is unlike nearly every other drug for unipolar depression since it does not block any monoamine transporter. Instead, mirtazapine is a multifunctional drug with five principal mechanisms of action: 5HT2A, 5HT2C, 5HT3, α2-adrenergic, and H1 histamine antagonism. The clinical consequences of blocking H1 receptors potentially result in sedation and weight gain. Blocking 5HT2A receptors leads to increases in downstream release of dopamine in the prefrontal cortex. 5HT2A antagonism also improves sleep, especially slow-wave sleep, which can be important in depression. Blocking 5HT2C receptors results in enhanced release of dopamine and norepinephrine (NE) in the prefrontal cortex, which may help in depression. Alpha-2 antagonism is another way to enhance the release of monoamines and exert an antidepressant action in unipolar depression. When an α2-antagonist is administered, norepinephrine can no longer turn off its own release, resulting in disinhibited noradrenergic neurons and increased NE. Alpha-2 antagonism also results in disinhibited serotonin release when NE migrates to the α2 presynaptic heteroreceptor on the serotonin neuron (Stahl, 2021) (See Figure 2.21C).

Vortioxetine

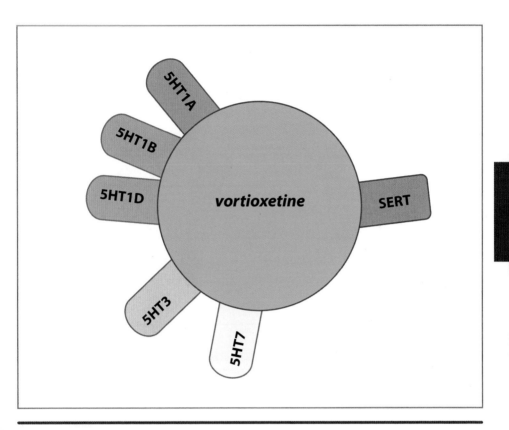

FIGURE 3.30. Vortioxetine, approved for treating unipolar depression, has multiple mechanisms of action. It causes SERT inhibition and has antagonist actions at 5HT3 and 5HT7 receptors. It also has agonist actions at 5HT1A receptors and weak partial agonist to antagonist actions at 5HT1B/D receptors. This unique blend of pharmacological actions leads to downstream release of many different neurotransmitters that result in antidepressant actions and pro-cognitive benefits (Stahl, 2015a). By combining SERT inhibition with 5HT1A agonist actions, these mechanisms alone are sufficient for antidepressant action, since they raise serotonin (5HT) levels, and the release of pro-cognitive neurotransmitters dopamine (DA), acetylcholine (ACh), and norepinephrine (NE). Additionally, when 5HT1 B/D presynaptic autoreceptors are blocked simultaneously, negative feedback to serotonin release cannot occur, so serotonin release increases further. Additional pro-cognitive actions of vortioxetine are potentially attributed to antagonist/ partial agonist actions on 5HT1B receptors located on the presynaptic nerve terminals of ACh, DA, histamine (H), and NE in the prefrontal cortex, disinhibiting their release (Stahl, 2015b). One of the most potent actions of vortioxetine is its 5HT3 antagonist properties, which enhances the release of pro-cognitive neurotransmitters ACh, DA, and NE. Finally, by blocking 5HT7 receptors, this results in enhanced 5HT release, especially in the presence of SERT inhibition. Thus, vortioxetine's pharmacological mechanism of action is multimodal, with numerous synergistic mechanisms resulting in antidepressant and pro-cognitive actions (Stahl, 2021).

Neuroactive Steroids

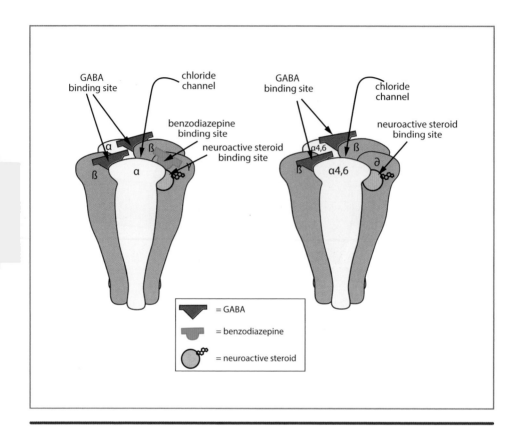

FIGURE 3.31. Neuroactive steroids bind to GABA$_A$ receptors at a specific allosteric site called the neuroactive steroid site, which enhances the inhibitory action of GABA at GABA$_A$ receptors. Neuroactive steroids target the benzodiazepine-sensitive GABA$_A$ receptors, similarly to benzodiazepines, but also the benzodiazepine-insensitive GABA$_A$ receptors, unlike benzodiazepines. Since benzodiazepines do not have antidepressant actions, it is the targeting of the benzodiazepine-insensitive GABA$_A$ receptors that is thought to be the primary mechanism of antidepressant action of neuroactive steroids (Belelli et al., 2020; Botella et al., 2017; Chen et al., 2019). The benzodiazepine-insensitive GABA$_A$ receptors are extrasynaptic and mediate tonic inhibition. When agents bind to these receptors, the result is rapid and possibly enduring antidepressant treatment; however, the full explanation of how this happens has not been elucidated. Targeting GABA action is a novel treatment for depression and comes from observations that GABA levels are reduced in the plasma, spinal fluid, and brains of depressed patients, and mRNA levels for the specific GABA$_A$ receptor subunits that encode the benzodiazepine-insensitive receptor subtypes are also deficient in the brains of depressed patients who died by suicide. Neuroactive steroids may compensate for these GABA-related deficits and may be how they mediate their rapid-onset antidepressant effects (Stahl, 2021) (See Figures 2.25 and 2.26).

Allopregnanolone

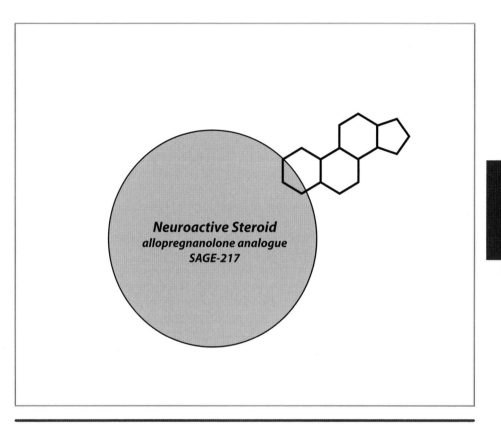

FIGURE 3.32. SAGE-217 (zuranolone) is a synthetic orally active allopregnanolone analogue in clinical testing as a rapid-onset oral antidepressant for major depressive disorder with some promising preliminary results (Lüscher and Möhler, 2019; Meltzer-Brody and Kanes, 2020). Another analogue of allopregnanolone, brexanolone, is also a neurosteroid and positive allosteric modulator at the GABA$_A$ receptor. It is FDA-approved and administered intravenously for the treatment of postpartum depression. Zuranolone has much better bioavailability than brexanolone and does not need to be administered intravenously. Zuranolone was granted Fast Track Designation by the FDA in 2017 for major depressive disorder (MDD) and Breakthrough Therapy Designation in 2018. In early 2022, zuranolone met the trial objectives of a phase 3 study (CORAL Study), demonstrating a rapid and statistically significant reduction in depressive symptoms at Day 3 and over the 2-week treatment period (Sage Therapeutics Press Release, Feb 2022).

Antidepressant Drugs for Bipolar Depression

A major paradigm shift is underway in the treatment of bipolar depression and depression with mixed features. The outdated perspective focused solely on the use of monoamine reuptake inhibitors as antidepressants for unipolar and bipolar depression. While many antidepressant agents contain monoamine reuptake inhibiting properties, current practice guidelines and United States Food and Drug Administration approvals are moving away from treatment of bipolar depression and depression with mixed features with the standard monoamine reuptake inhibitors that are so commonly used for the treatment of unipolar depression. There is increasing reservation about the use of reuptake inhibitors for patients who have depression with mixed features and for patients with bipolar depression. For these patients, these agents should instead be used as second-line treatments to augment other agents. As best practice evolves for treating bipolar depression and depression with mixed features, first-line treatment is now one of the specifically approved serotonin/dopamine blockers, and not a monoamine reuptake inhibitor. There remains plenty of controversy over this recommendation, as many prescribers still advocate for monoamine reuptake inhibitors in some patients with bipolar depression. However, growing research demonstrates failure of monoamine reuptake inhibiting agents to work consistently in bipolar depression or in mixed features. Additionally, these drugs can induce intolerable activating side effects, including manic episodes and even suicidality in patients with bipolar/mixed depression. In this next section, we will address evidence-based agents for bipolar depression by class: serotonin/dopamine blockers, "mood stabilizers," and anticonvulsants, along with combination treatments.

Serotonin/Dopamine Blocker: Olanzapine-Fluoxetine

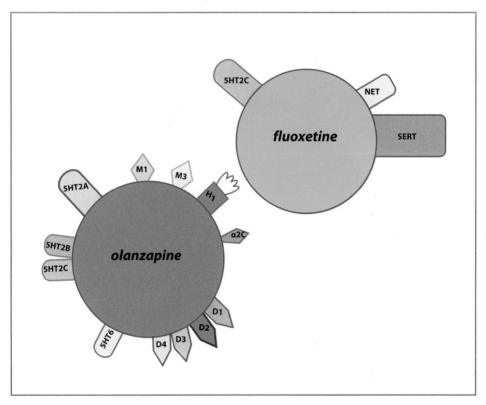

FIGURE 3.33. Olanzapine-fluoxetine combination is approved for bipolar depression, in addition to bipolar mania and unipolar depression. The antidepressant action is likely linked to its 5HT2A and 5HT2C antagonist properties. The D2 antagonism may theoretically also prevent mania (Stahl, 2021).

Serotonin/Dopamine Blocker: Quetiapine

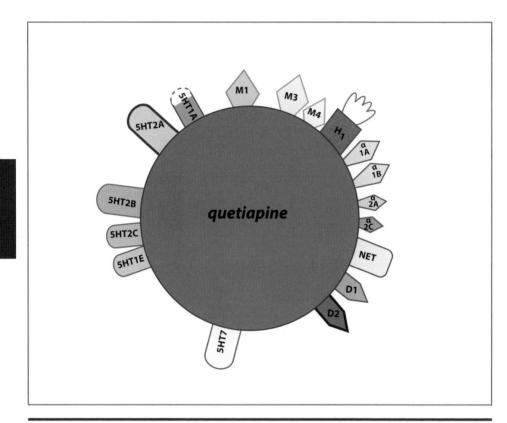

FIGURE 3.34. Quetiapine is approved for bipolar depression, bipolar mania, and as an augmenting agent with SSRIs/SNRIs for treatment-resistant unipolar depression. Its antidepressant mechanisms involve the combined actions of quetiapine and its active metabolite norquetiapine at both 5HT2C receptors and at the norepinephrine transporter (NET). It also has antidepressant effects as an antagonist at the 5HT2A receptor, 5HT7 receptor, and α2A receptor, in addition to agonist action at the 5HT1A receptor (Stahl, 2021).

Serotonin/Dopamine Blocker: Lurasidone

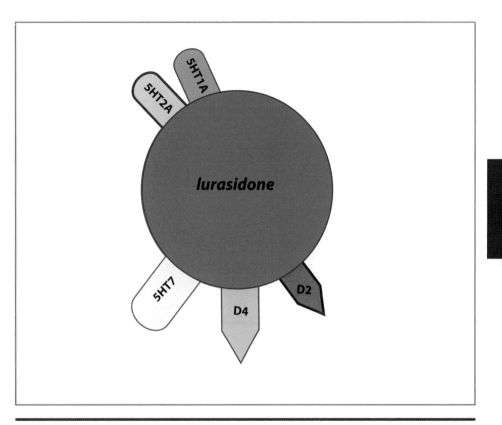

FIGURE 3.35. Lurasidone has several hypothetical antidepressant receptor binding properties: blockade of 5HT2A, 5HT7, and α2 receptors with agonist actions at 5HT1A receptors. Post hoc analysis of lurasidone in bipolar depression revealed that patients with mixed features respond as well as patients without mixed features (Suppes et al., 2016). More importantly, lurasidone is the only drug to be studied in a large, randomized multicenter trial of unipolar depression with mixed features and to demonstrate robust antidepressant efficacy in these patients without inducing mania. Lurasidone is approved for bipolar depression and is prescribed at lower doses than those used for the treatment of psychosis in schizophrenia and is generally well tolerated with little tendency for weight gain or metabolic disturbances. It is one of the most widely prescribed agents for bipolar depression (Stahl, 2021).

Serotonin/Dopamine Blocker: Cariprazine

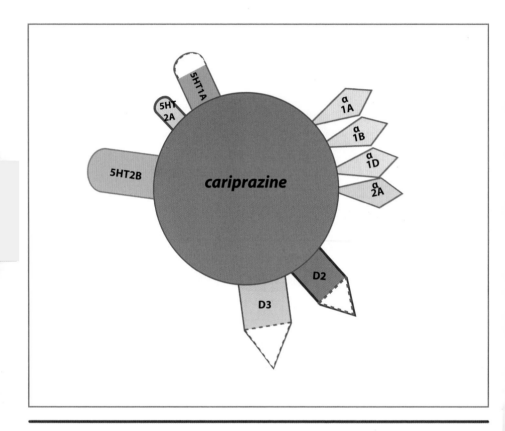

FIGURE 3.36. Cariprazine is a D3/D2/5HT1A partial agonist approved for the treatment of bipolar depression and acute bipolar mania, with ongoing trials as an adjunct to SSRIs/SNRIs in unipolar depression. Cariprazine has 5HT1A partial agonist actions as well as α2 antagonist actions, each with potential antidepressant mechanisms. What sets cariprazine apart from other agents in this class of serotonin/dopamine antagonist/partial agonists is its unique highly potent action at D3 dopamine receptors as a partial agonist. Cariprazine is more potent than dopamine at the D3 receptor and the most potent of any available agent at the D3 receptor. In this way, cariprazine can compete with dopamine for the D3 receptor. Presynaptic actions of D3 antagonism/partial agonism in the ventral tegmental area (VTA) most likely contribute to cariprazine's antidepressant actions. When D3 antagonists/partial agonists act in the VTA to block them, this disinhibits the dopamine neurons projecting to the prefrontal cortex and they release dopamine onto D1 receptors, resulting in antidepressant effects (Stahl et al., 2020; Stahl, 2021).

Serotonin/Dopamine Blocker: Lumateperone

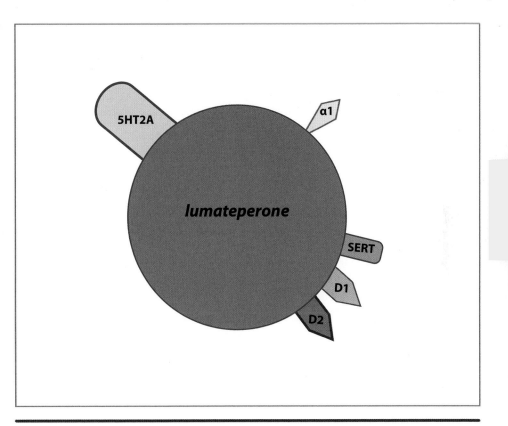

FIGURE 3.37. Lumateperone has very high affinity for the 5HT2A receptor, moderate affinity for the D2, D1, and α1 receptor, and low affinity for the H1 receptors. Lumateperone also has affinity for the serotonin transporter (SERT), which is likely to contribute to its antidepressant effects. It recently received FDA approval for bipolar depression. The approval was based on two positive phase 3 placebo-controlled studies that demonstrated efficacy in improving depressive symptoms in patients with bipolar I and bipolar II, both as monotherapy and as adjunctive therapy with lithium or valproate. Lumateperone has also demonstrated favorable safety and tolerability (Stahl, 2021; Zhang and Hendrick, 2018).

"Mood Stabilizers" for Depression-Minded Treatments

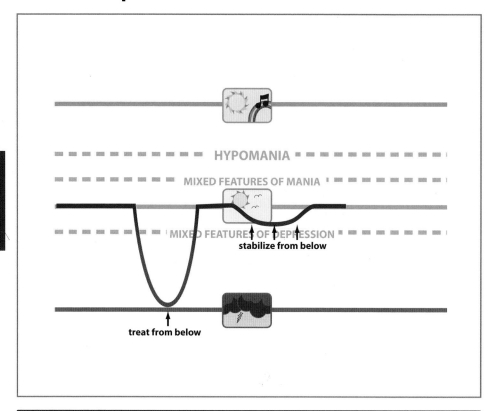

FIGURE 3.38. Although the ideal "mood stabilizer" would treat bipolar depression and mania while also preventing episodes of either pole, in reality different agents may be efficacious for different phases of bipolar disorder. Some agents may be "depression-minded" and thus able to "treat from below" and/or "stabilize from below." The purpose of these drugs is to prevent the symptoms of bipolar depression (Stahl, 2021).

"Mood Stabilizers": Lithium

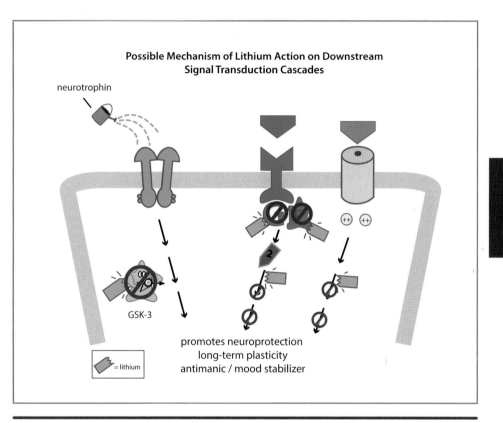

Possible Mechanism of Lithium Action on Downstream Signal Transduction Cascades

neurotrophin

GSK-3

= lithium

promotes neuroprotection
long-term plasticity
antimanic / mood stabilizer

FIGURE 3.39. While lithium is most well known for its efficacy in treating mania in bipolar disorder, it is also used to treat depressive episodes in bipolar disorder and as an augmenting agent to drugs for depression in treatment-resistant depression, but it is not formally approved for these uses. While it is the oldest treatment for bipolar disorder, its mechanism of action is not completely understood. Several potential mechanisms exist and are depicted here. Lithium's therapeutic actions may work by affecting signal transduction, potentially through its inhibition of second-messenger enzymes such as inositol monophosphatase (right), by modulation of G-proteins (middle), or downstream signal transduction cascades, including glycogen synthase kinase 3 (GSK-3) (left) (Chiu and Chuang, 2010; Stahl, 2021).

Anticonvulsants as "Mood Stabilizers" for Bipolar Depression

The use of anticonvulsants as "mood stabilizers" has been utilized for the treatment of both mania and depression in bipolar disorder for quite some time. However, these agents would be better classified for their pharmacological mechanism of action at ion channels rather than as "mood stabilizers" or "anticonvulsants." Because the known anticonvulsants carbamazepine and valproate proved effective in treating the manic phase of bipolar disorder, this led to the concept that any anticonvulsant would be a mood stabilizer; however, this has not proven to be the case. Anticonvulsants have a variety of different mechanisms.

Anticonvulsants as "Mood Stabilizers": Lamotrigine

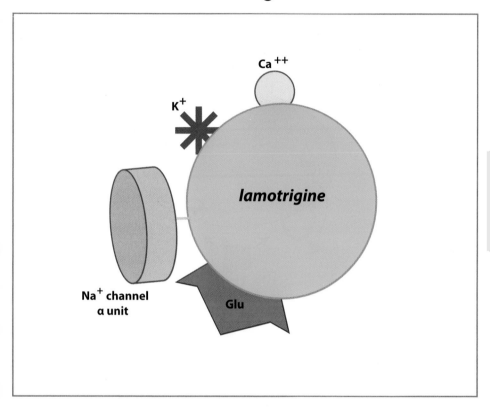

FIGURE 3.40. Lamotrigine is approved as a "mood stabilizer" but has very different therapeutic actions than other mood stabilizers, such as valproate and carbamazepine. While the FDA has not approved lamotrigine for acute bipolar depression, most experts believe that it is effective in treating bipolar depression. Lamotrigine has been approved to prevent recurrence of both depression and mania in bipolar disorder. The medication may work by blocking the alpha subunit of voltage-sensitive sodium channels (VSSCs) and could perhaps have actions at other ion channels for calcium and potassium. Lamotrigine is thought to reduce the release of the excitatory neurotransmitter glutamate. It is unclear whether this action is secondary to blocking the activation of VSSCs or to some additional synaptic action. Reducing excitatory glutamatergic neurotransmission, especially if excessive during bipolar depression, may be a unique mechanism of action of lamotrigine and explain why it has such a different clinical profile as a treatment from below and a stabilizer from below for bipolar depression (Stahl, 2021).

Anticonvulsants as "Mood Stabilizers":
Valproate

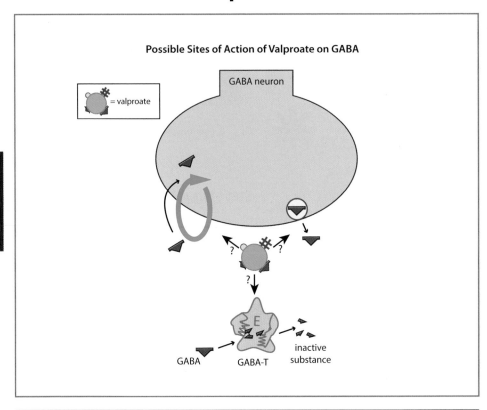

Possible Sites of Action of Valproate on GABA

FIGURE 3.41. For all anticonvulsants, the exact mechanism of action is uncertain; however, even less is understood about the mechanism of action for valproic acid, or valproate, compared to other anticonvulsants. Valproate may work by interfering with voltage-sensitive sodium channels, enhancing the inhibitory actions of gamma-aminobutyric acid (GABA), and regulating downstream signal transduction cascades, although which of these actions may be related to mood stabilization is unclear. Valproate may also interact with other ion channels, such as voltage-sensitive calcium channels, and also indirectly block glutamate (Glu) actions. Antidepressant actions of valproate have not been well established, nor has it been shown to convincingly stabilize against recurrent depressive episodes, but there may be some efficacy for the depressed phase of bipolar disorder in some patients (Stahl, 2021).

Combinations for Bipolar Depression

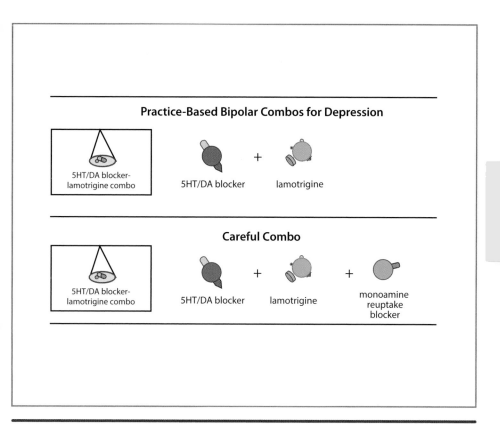

FIGURE 3.42. Most patients with bipolar disorder will require treatment with two or more agents. Combinations that are not well studied in controlled trials, but that have some practice-based evidence for depression, include a serotonin/dopamine antagonist plus lamotrigine. Although controversial, some clinicians add a monoamine reuptake inhibitor to a serotonin/dopamine antagonist for bipolar depression. This is depicted here as a "Careful Combo" (Stahl, 2021).

Antidepressants for Mixed Depression

There are currently no agents approved for depression with mixed features. The small number of studies that have been conducted suggest poor responses to monoamine reuptake inhibitors, and a growing body of evidence suggests that certain serotonin/dopamine blockers, particularly those already approved for bipolar depression, are the preferred treatment method for mixed features.

Lurasidone for Mixed Depression

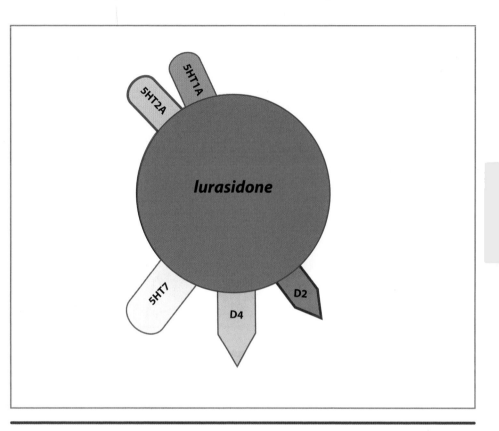

FIGURE 3.43. Lurasidone is prescribed for bipolar depression and for mixed features in doses lower than those generally used to treat psychosis. Lurasidone is the only agent to be studied in a large, randomized multicenter trial of unipolar depression with mixed features and to demonstrate robust antidepressant efficacy in these patients without inducing mania (Suppes et al., 2016). Lurasidone has several hypothetical antidepressant receptor binding properties: blockade of 5HT2A, 5HT7, and α2 receptors with agonist actions at 5HT1A receptors. It is one of the only agents to demonstrate on post hoc analysis of bipolar depression that those with bipolar depression and mixed features respond as well to lurasidone as patients with bipolar depression without mixed features.

Cariprazine for Mixed Depression

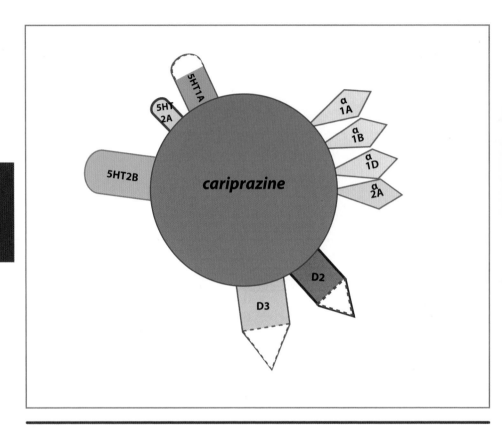

FIGURE 3.44. Cariprazine is a D3/D2/5HT1A partial agonist approved for acute bipolar depression and acute bipolar mania. Post hoc analysis has shown significant clinical improvement both in mania with mixed features of depression and bipolar depression with mixed features of mania (Stahl et al., 2020). Cariprazine has some of the most robust and wide-ranging efficacy known across the entire bipolar spectrum (Stahl et al., 2020; Stahl, 2021).

Lumateperone for Mixed Depression

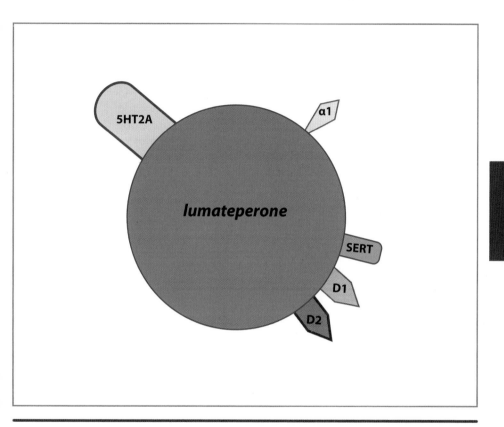

FIGURE 3.45. Lumateperone has very high affinity for the 5HT2A receptor, moderate affinity for the D2, D1, and α1 receptor, and low affinity for the H1 receptors. It is approved for the treatment of depressive episodes associated with bipolar I or bipolar II disorder. A post hoc analysis of the phase 3 study the approval was based on revealed statistically significant reductions in depressive symptoms and disease severity, as measured by Montgomery-Asberg Depression Rating Scale (MADRS) total score and Clinical Global Impression-Bipolar-Severity (CGI-BP-S) total score, in groups with and without mixed features (McIntyre et al., Submitted 2022). Results suggest that lumateperone may be effective as treatment for bipolar depression with mixed features.

Drugs for Mania in Bipolar Disorder and Mixed Features

When D2 antagonists were approved for schizophrenia, it was not surprising that these agents would be effective in treating psychotic symptoms associated with mania, since D2 blockers are used to treat psychosis in general. However, dopamine/serotonin blockers have been effective in treating the core nonpsychotic symptoms of mania, as well as for maintenance treatment to prevent the recurrence of mania. Positron emission tomography (PET) scans of patients with mania show the same excessive presynaptic dopamine levels and release in mesostriatal dopamine neurons in acute bipolar mania as for acute psychosis in schizophrenia (Stahl, 2017). Thus, blocking excessive dopamine at D2 receptors should have as much of an antimanic effect in bipolar mania as it has an antipsychotic effect in schizophrenia. However, not all agents in the serotonin/dopamine blocker class approved to treat schizophrenia are also approved to treat acute bipolar mania, and not all of those approved for acute bipolar mania are approved for bipolar maintenance. Differences in receptor binding profiles could explain why some agents are approved in mania and others are not. To enhance antimanic response and to prevent relapse into manic episodes, lithium and valproate are commonly utilized in conjunction with those dopamine/serotonin blockers approved for the treatment of mania (Stahl, 2021).

Serotonin/Dopamine Blockers for Mania

	Evidence of efficacy in mixed features	FDA-approved for bipolar mania	FDA-approved for bipolar maintenance
Cariprazine	Yes, MMX, DMX	Yes	
Quetiapine	Yes, MMX	Yes	Yes
Olanzapine	Yes, MMX	Yes	Yes
Aripiprazole		Yes	Yes
Asenapine	Yes, MMX	Yes	Yes
Risperidone		Yes	Yes
Ziprasidone	Yes, MMX	Yes	Yes

MMX, mania with mixed features; DMX, depression with mixed features

FIGURE 3.46. There are several serotonin/dopamine blockers that are effective, and many are approved for treating mania in bipolar disorder. The chart summarizes which ones are approved, which have demonstrated efficacy in mixed features, and which are approved for bipolar maintenance (Stahl, 2021).

"Mood Stabilizers" for Mania-Minded Treatments

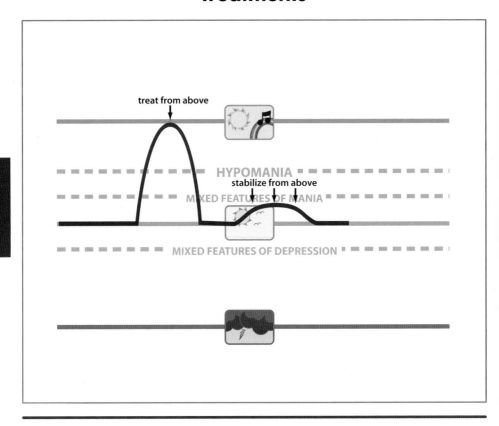

FIGURE 3.47. Some mood-stabilizing agents may be "mania-minded" and "treat from above," meaning they are able to "stabilize from above" or reduce and/or prevent symptoms of mania (Stahl, 2021).

Lithium for Mania in Bipolar Disorder

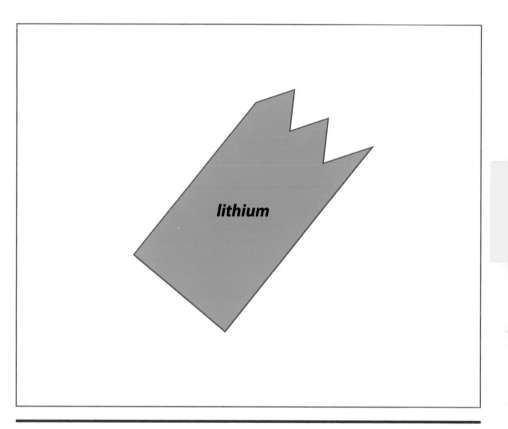

FIGURE 3.48. Bipolar mania has classically been treated with lithium for over 50 years. Lithium is an ion with a mechanism of action that is not completely understood. Various signal transduction sites beyond neurotransmitter receptors are most likely involved. This includes second messengers such as the phosphatidyl inositol system, where lithium inhibits the enzyme inositol monophosphatase, modulation of G-proteins, and, most recently, regulation of gene expression for growth factors and neuronal plasticity by interaction with downstream signal transduction cascades, including inhibition of GSK-3 (glycogen synthase kinase 3) and protein kinase C. Lithium has been proven effective in manic episodes, and in maintenance of recurrence, especially for manic episodes (Chiu and Chuang, 2010; Stahl, 2021).

Valproate for Mania in Bipolar Disorder

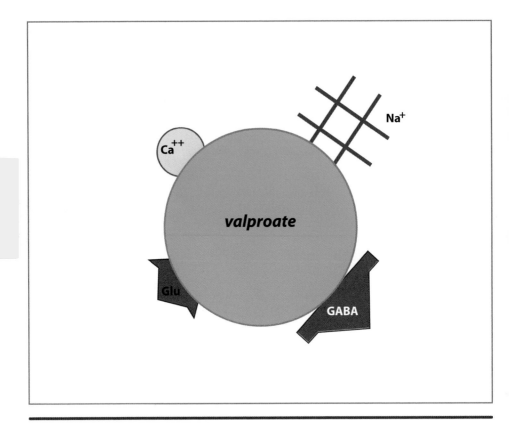

FIGURE 3.49. This simple molecule has multiple and complex clinical effects, and research is trying to determine which of the various mechanisms explain the "mood-stabilizing" antimanic effects. One hypothesis is that valproate acts to diminish excessive neurotransmission by diminishing the flow of ions through voltage-sensitive sodium channels (VSSCs). No specific molecular site of action for valproate has been identified but it's possible that valproate may change the sensitivity of sodium channels by altering phosphorylation of sodium channels, either by binding directly to the VSSC or its regulatory units, or by inhibiting phosphorylating enzymes. If less sodium is able to pass into neurons, this could theoretically result in diminished release of glutamate and thus less excitatory neurotransmission. Other potential mechanisms are that valproate enhances gamma-aminobutyric acid (GABA) actions, or that valproate regulates downstream signal transduction cascades (Stahl, 2021).

Carbamazepine for Mania in Bipolar Disorder

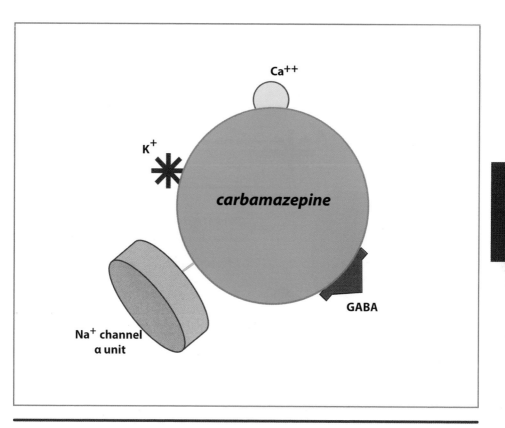

FIGURE 3.50. Carbamazepine was the first agent shown to be effective in the manic phase of bipolar disorder; however, it did not receive US FDA approval until recently with a once-daily controlled-release formulation. Carbamazepine is hypothesized to act by blocking voltage-sensitive sodium channels (VSSCs), potentially at a site within the channel itself, also known as the α subunit of VSSCs. Carbamazepine has profound immediate suppressant effects upon the bone marrow, requiring initial monitoring of blood counts, and notable induction of the cytochrome P450 enzyme 3A4 (Stahl, 2021).

Lamotrigine for Mania in Bipolar Disorder

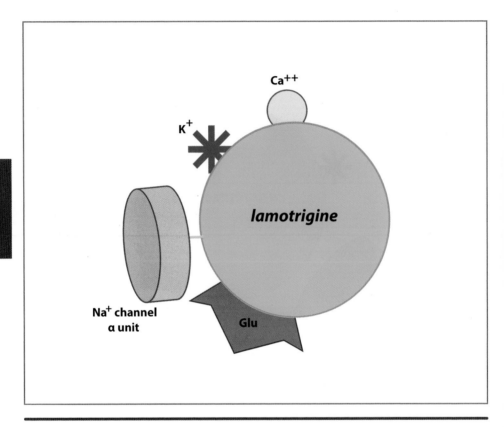

FIGURE 3.51. Lamotrigine is approved as a "mood stabilizer," however it is not approved for acute mania. It is approved to prevent recurrence of both mania and depression in bipolar disorder. It is possible that lamotrigine reduces glutamate release through its blockade of voltage-sensitive sodium channels (VSSCs). Alternatively, it may have this effect via an additional synaptic action that has not yet been identified (Stahl, 2021).

Combinations for Bipolar Mania

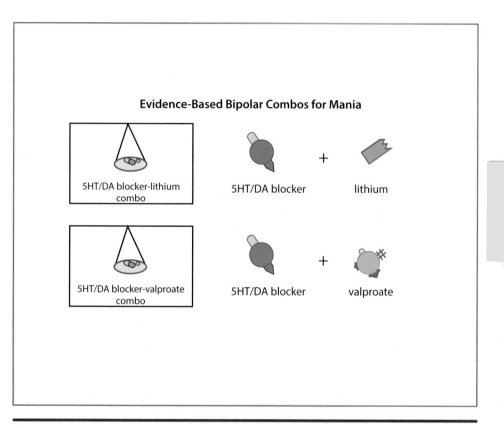

Evidence-Based Bipolar Combos for Mania

5HT/DA blocker-lithium combo	5HT/DA blocker + lithium
5HT/DA blocker-valproate combo	5HT/DA blocker + valproate

FIGURE 3.52. Most patients with bipolar disorder will require treatment with two or more agents. The combinations with the most evidence for mania include the addition of a serotonin/dopamine antagonist to either lithium or valproate (Stahl, 2021).

Treatment Resistance in Depressive Disorders

Remission—the resolution of essentially all symptoms—is the initial goal when treating patients with depression. Approximately one-third to one-half of depressed patients will remit during the first trial with any antidepressant (Little, 2009; Saveanu, 2015). Unfortunately, for those who fail to remit the likelihood of remission with another antidepressant monotherapy decreases with each successive trial. For example, in STAR*D, after a year of treatment with four sequential antidepressants taken for 12 weeks each, only two-thirds of patients achieved remission (Rush et al., 2006).

Patients who do not achieve remission not only experience ongoing impairment despite treatment, but are also at increased risk for full relapse compared to those who do remit (Judd et al., 1998; Rush et al., 2006).

It is very important for patients to achieve remission as early in the treatment course as possible; however, there may be impediments to achieving early remission. Strategies to optimize outcomes for patients potentially include combining mechanisms earlier in the course of treatment, prompt attention to specific residual symptoms, communication about and strategies to address side effects, and consideration of "wellness" factors beyond mere symptom resolution.

In this chapter, we discuss these strategies, along with augmentation, switching strategies, and the addition of nonpharmacological adjunctive treatments for unipolar depression. We also address treatment-resistant strategies and adjunctive treatments in bipolar disorder.

Impediments to Remission: Anxiety and Residual Symptoms

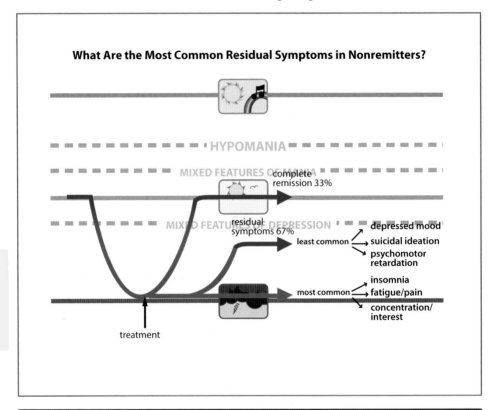

What Are the Most Common Residual Symptoms in Nonremitters?

HYPOMANIA

MIXED FEATURES OF MANIA

complete remission 33%

MIXED FEATURES OF DEPRESSION

residual symptoms 67%

least common

depressed mood
suicidal ideation
psychomotor retardation

most common

insomnia
fatigue/pain
concentration/interest

treatment

FIGURE 4.1. Some of the strongest impediments to remission are residual symptoms. The most common symptoms that persist after antidepressant treatment, thus preventing remission, are insomnia, fatigue and painful physical complaints, cognitive problems such as trouble concentrating, and lack of interest or motivation (Stahl, 2021). These particular symptoms present 94% of the time during a depressive episode and persist 44% of the time between depressive episodes (Conradi et al., 2011). In contrast, antidepressants appear to work fairly well in improving depressed mood, suicidal ideation, and psychomotor retardation (Stahl, 2021). Residual symptoms are often predictive of poor long-term outcomes, including increased disability, more frequent relapses, relationship and work difficulties, and suicide. Additionally, more severe anxiety at baseline is associated with lower remission rates, independent of depression severity or diagnostic comorbidity (Saveanu et al., 2015).

Monitoring Treatment: Time Course of Most Antidepressants

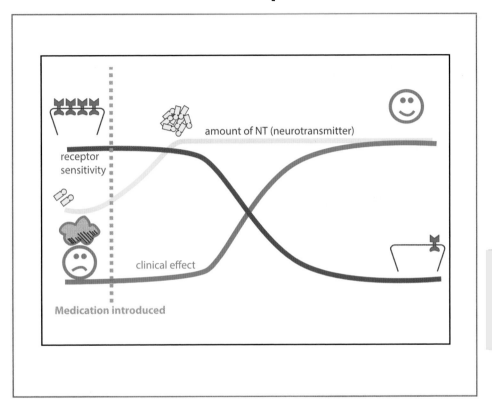

amount of NT (neurotransmitter)

receptor sensitivity

clinical effect

Medication introduced

FIGURE 4.2. While typical antidepressants increase monoamines almost immediately, the clinical improvement in depression may be delayed for weeks. This can be challenging for patients, and often leads to nonadherence (Gartlehner et al., 2005). The temporal correlation of clinical effects with alterations in receptor sensitivity has given rise to the hypothesis that changes in neurotransmitter receptor sensitivity may actually mediate the clinical effects of antidepressants. These clinical effects involve antidepressant and anxiolytic actions in addition to the development of tolerance to the acute side effects. Throughout the course of antidepressant treatment, monitoring patients by using brief, standardized tools can help to identify patients at risk for relapse or nonadherence (Rost, 2009). Studies suggest that tools such as mood-tracking apps can be integrated fairly easily into clinical practice (Duffy et al., 2008). Additionally, defining and assessing therapeutic endpoints specific to the individual patient provides a good measure of treatment effects (Trivedi, 2009).

Common and Troubling Side Effects

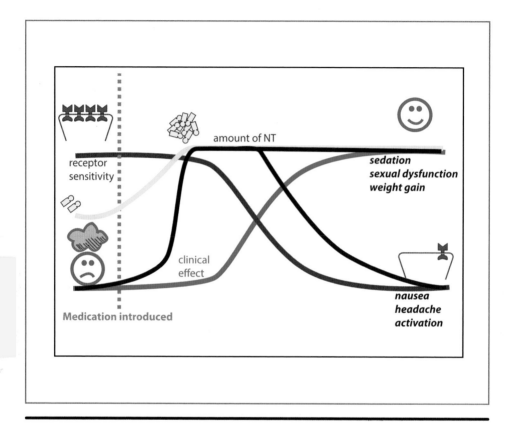

FIGURE 4.3. While the clinical effects of antidepressants do not occur for several weeks, side effects can often be immediate, posing additional problems for adherence. The delay in the therapeutic effects of antidepressants is hypothesized to occur because the initial increase in monoamines leads to downstream alterations in gene expression. In contrast, the acute onset of common side effects such as nausea and headache may be linked directly to rapid changes in neurotransmitter levels following antidepressant induction (Bostwick, 2010; Stahl, 2021). These side effects tend to be short lived, which may be explained by downstream receptor sensitivity (Stahl, 2021). Appropriate and prompt management of side effects is essential in order to improve adherence and maximize the potential for successful treatment.

Mechanisms Associated With Short-Term Side Effects

	Nausea	Headache	Activation
5HT reuptake inhibition	X	X	X
NE reuptake inhibition	X		X
DA reuptake inhibition			Psychomotor
5HT2C antagonism			X

FIGURE 4.4. In the short term, some of the most troubling side effects are nausea, headache, and activation (Bostwick, 2010; Cascade et al., 2009; Kelly et al., 2008). Nausea may occur with 5HT reuptake inhibitors because the increase in synaptic 5HT leads to stimulation of 5HT3 receptors. 5HT3 receptors that are localized in the chemoreceptor trigger zone of the brainstem mediate nausea and vomiting, while 5HT3 receptors in the gastrointestinal tract mediate nausea, vomiting, and bowel motility. Management strategies to alleviate nausea include slower titration, divided dosing, taking the dose with food, and consuming ginger. A selective 5HT3 antagonist, such as ondansetron, tropisetron, or granisetron, can be used to relieve treatment-induced nausea (Stahl, 2021).

Headache is also a common side effect of serotonergic antidepressants and may be related to downstream actions at 5HT2 receptors (Srikiatkhachorn, 2001). Headache is generally best managed by over-the-counter pain relievers; however, avoid combining serotonergic drugs with anticoagulants (e.g., nonsteroidal anti-inflammatory drugs or NSAIDs) due to the potential for increased risk of bleeding. Slower titration may also be beneficial.

Mechanisms Associated With Long-Term Side Effects

	Sexual Dysfunction	Weight Gain	Sedation
5HT reuptake inhibition	X	X	
5HT2 antagonism	Indirect	X	
Alpha 1 antagonism	X	X	X
Histamine 1 antagonism		X	X
Anti-cholinergic	X	X	
NOS inhibition	X		

FIGURE 4.5. In the long term, the most troubling side effects are sexual dysfunction, weight gain, and sedation (Bostwick, 2010; Cascade et al., 2009; Kelly et al., 2008). Presumably, 5HT has a negative impact on sexual function because it can reduce dopamine (DA) neurotransmission downstream by stimulating 5HT2A and 5HT2C receptors (Morehouse et al., 2011). Other potential mechanisms for sexual dysfunction include the anticholinergic effects and alpha-1 adrenergic receptor blocking effects of some antidepressants. Selecting agents that are 5HT2A antagonists such as trazodone, mirtazapine, and vortioxetine may be less likely to cause sexual side effects. Regular exercise can also improve sexual function (Lorenz and Meston, 2014).

Weight gain is an intolerable side effect for many patients. Medication-induced weight gain may be associated with antagonism of 5HT2C receptors in the hypothalamus, where appetite is largely regulated. All patients prescribed an antidepressant should be monitored for weight, appetite, and metabolic changes. Diet and exercise guidance should be offered, and potential switching or augmentation strategies to reduce weight gain should be considered.

Sedation is most common with agents that have secondary properties of alpha 1 antagonism and/or histamine 1 antagonism, such as many tricyclic antidepressants (Morehouse et al., 2011; Stahl, 2021). Adjusting dosing to correspond with sleep time may improve symptoms. Increasing daytime exercise, using adjunctive medications, or switching to a non-sedative antidepressant can relieve sedation symptoms.

Treatment-Resistant Strategies for Unipolar Depression

Treatment responses are not "all or none" phenomena. Genetic testing has the potential of assisting with the selection of psychotropic drug treatment for depression, especially when several first-line treatments have failed to work or to be tolerated. It is possible to obtain, from various laboratories, genetic variants for a number of genes that regulate drug metabolism and hypothetically regulate efficacy and side effects of drugs in depression. Utilizing pharmacogenetic testing in addition to measuring drug plasma levels will improve the optimization of treatment and accelerate the development of individualized treatment plans. With treatment-resistant unipolar depression, understanding potential augmentation strategies and switching strategies can be incredibly helpful in optimizing overall clinical outcome for individual patients. While genetic testing and plasma level testing can aid in these decisions, we limit our discussion here to evidence-based augmentation and switching strategies for treatment-resistant depression (TRD).

Augmentation Strategies:
Serotonin/Dopamine Blockers

Drug	Mechanism of Action	FDA-Approved for MDD
Aripiprazole	D2/5HT1A partial agonist	Yes (adjunct)
Olanzapine-fluoxetine	D2/5HT2A/5HT2C antagonist/NET/SERT	Yes (together)
Quetiapine	D2/5HT2C/NET/ 5HT2A/5HT7/α2A	Yes (adjunct)
Brexpiprazole	D2/5HT1A partial agonist/5HT2A antagonist/α1 antagonist	Yes (adjunct)
Cariprazine	D3/D2/5HT1A partial agonist/5HT2A/α1/α2 antagonist	No
Lumateperone	5HT2A/D2/D1/ α1antagonist/SERT inhibitor	No

FIGURE 4.6. Serotonin/dopamine blockers originally developed for psychosis are now some of the most common adjunctive treatments to SSRIs/SNRIs in patients with unipolar depression who fail to respond adequately to one or more trials of the various first-line monoamine agents previously discussed. This chart summarizes the most evidence-based agents in this category for treatment-resistant unipolar depression: olanzapine-fluoxetine, quetiapine, aripiprazole, brexpiprazole, cariprazine, and lumateperone. Olanzapine-fluoxetine combination is a potent SERT/5HT2C inhibitor and highly efficacious for treatment-resistant depression (TRD) (Stahl, 2021).

Of these agents, cariprazine, olanzapine-fluoxetine, and quetiapine are approved for bipolar depression; lurasidone is also approved. Several of these agents are approved for mania and as adjunctive treatment for major depressive disorder (MDD). While many of the same agents that are approved for bipolar depression demonstrate efficacy for mixed features, there are currently no agents that are approved for mixed depression (Suppes et al., 2016; Stahl, 2021).

Augmentation Strategies: Ketamine

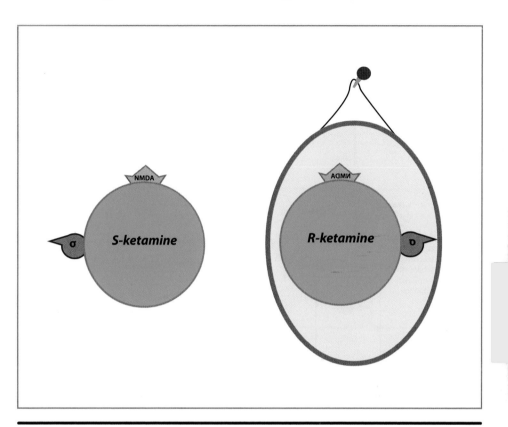

FIGURE 4.7. There is a growing body of research on the use of intravenous ketamine to effectively treat depression in patients who have not responded to monoamine therapy. Ketamine is an approved anesthetic but used off-label for treatment-resistant depression (Aan het Rot M et al., 2010; Ibrahim et al., 2012; Murrough et al., 2013). Intravenous ketamine is a racemic mixture of R- and S-ketamine which acts as an NMDA receptor antagonist, with additional weak receptor actions at the sigma-1 receptor, the norepinephrine transporter (NET), μ-opioid receptors, and the serotonin reuptake transporter (SERT). What is unique about ketamine infusions, is the rapid, almost immediate onset of antidepressant effects. The S enantiomer of ketamine is approved for treatment-resistant depression in an intranasal formulation for administration and is called esketamine. The specific pharmacology of R- versus S-ketamine and their active metabolites is still being determined in terms of neurotrophic actions. However, esketamine is active as an acute rapid-onset antidepressant (Wajs et al., 2020). It is administered intranasally and rapidly, so that longer intravenous infusions are not necessary. After twice-weekly initiation, esketamine can be given intranasally in weekly or biweekly dosing as an augmenting agent to standard drugs for depression.

Ketamine: Mechanism of Action

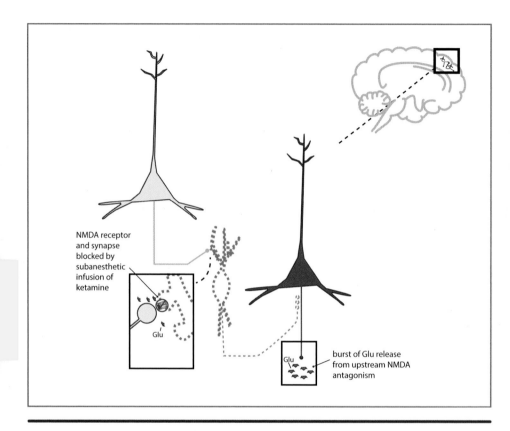

FIGURE 4.8. Ketamine's antidepressant effects seem to work via an immediate burst of downstream glutamate release after blocking NMDA receptors. Depicted here are two cortical glutamatergic pyramidal neurons and a GABAergic interneuron. If an NMDA receptor on a GABAergic interneuron is blocked by ketamine, this prevents the excitatory actions of glutamate (Glu) there. As a result, the GABA neuron is inactivated and can no longer inhibit the second cortical glutamatergic pyramidal neuron, resulting in a burst of glutamate from this second neuron. Glutamate activity heavily modulates synaptic potentiation via NMDA and AMPA receptor signaling. One hypothesis is that blockade of the NMDA receptor leads to rapid activation of AMPA, which triggers ERK/AKT signal transduction cascade, which then triggers the mammalian target of rapamycin (mTOR) pathway (Li et al., 2010; Stahl, 2013a). This in turn would lead to rapid AMPA-mediated synaptic potentiation and increase dendritic spine formation. Traditional antidepressants also cause synaptic potentiation; however, they do so through downstream alterations in intracellular signaling. This difference in mechanism of action may be what underlies ketamine's rapid antidepressant effects (Stahl, 2021).

Other Drug Combinations for Treatment-Resistant Depression

Other options to augment monoamine treatments for unipolar depression include agents that do not have robust antidepressant actions as monotherapies but can improve the action of the monoamine treatments (e.g., lithium, buspirone, and thyroid), as well as the popular and effective strategy of combining two monoamine drugs, each approved for unipolar depression, to create pharmacological synergy. However, none of these combinations are specifically approved.

While lithium is one of the most utilized treatments for mania, it has also been used for treatment-resistant unipolar depression. Lithium augmentation of monoamine reuptake inhibitors, particularly the classic tricyclic antidepressants, has been used in the past to boost treatment response in unipolar depression. Lithium is administered in doses lower than those used for mania but has fallen out of favor in recent years.

Buspirone is a 5HT1A partial agonist. Combining it with an SSRI/SNRI is another augmenting strategy for treatment-resistant depression. Administering drugs that have 5HT1A agonist actions is a preferred approach for augmenting SSRIs/SNRIs but using buspirone for this is less common today than using other agents with 5HT1A properties.

Abnormalities in thyroid hormone levels have long been associated with depression, and various forms and doses of thyroid hormones have for many years been utilized as augmenting agents to drugs for depression to either boost their efficacy in patients with inadequate response or to speed up their onset of action. Augmentation of treatments for either unipolar or bipolar depression with thyroid hormones has also fallen out of favor in recent years.

Combination therapies to boost neurotransmitter levels can be powerfully effective. The most common ones involve combining an SSRI with an NDRI or combining an SNRI with an NDRI. Combination strategies can also be effective at reducing unwanted side effects.

Triple-Action Combos

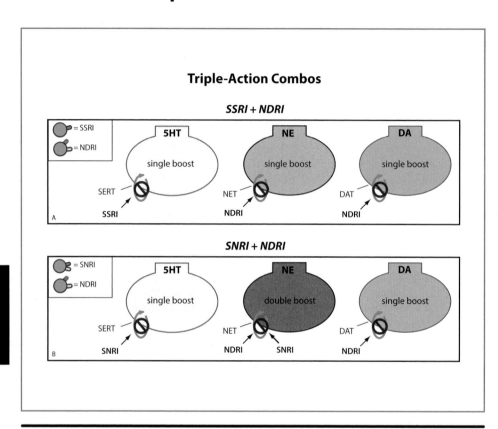

FIGURE 4.9. Triple-action (i.e., serotonin, dopamine, and norepinephrine) drugs for depression therapy with modulation of all three monoamines would be predicted to occur by combining either a selective serotonin reuptake inhibitor (SSRI) with a norepinephrine-dopamine reuptake inhibitor (NDRI) or combining a serotonin-norepinephrine reuptake inhibitor (SNRI) with a NDRI, providing even more noradrenergic and dopaminergic action. These are potentially the most popular combinations of two drugs for depression utilized in the United States. A) SSRI plus a NDRI leads to a single boost for serotonin (5HT), norepinephrine (NE), and dopamine (DA). B) SNRI plus a NDRI leads to a single boost for 5HT, a double boost for NE, and a single boost for DA (Stahl, 2021).

California Rocket Fuel

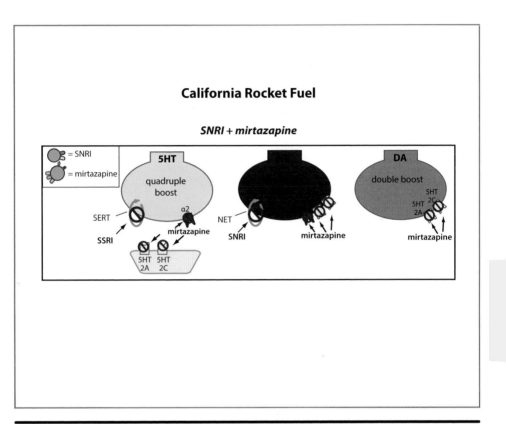

California Rocket Fuel

SNRI + mirtazapine

FIGURE 4.10. This powerfully potent combination capitalizes on the pharmacological synergy attained by adding the enhanced serotonin and norepinephrine release from inhibition of both serotonin and norepinephrine reuptake by an SNRI to the disinhibition of both serotonin and norepinephrine release by the α antagonist actions of mirtazapine. It is even possible that additional pro-dopaminergic actions result from the combination of norepinephrine reuptake blockade in the prefrontal cortex due to SNRIs with 5HT2C actions of mirtazapine disinhibiting dopamine release. This combination can provide very powerful antidepressant action for some patients with unipolar major depressive episodes (Stahl, 2021).

In a recent systematic review and meta-analysis, data collected from 38 randomized clinical trials (RCTs) revealed that combination of a monoamine reuptake inhibitor and an α2 antagonist was associated with superior outcomes relative to monotherapy, even when applied as first-line treatment (Henssler et al., 2022).

Arousal Combinations

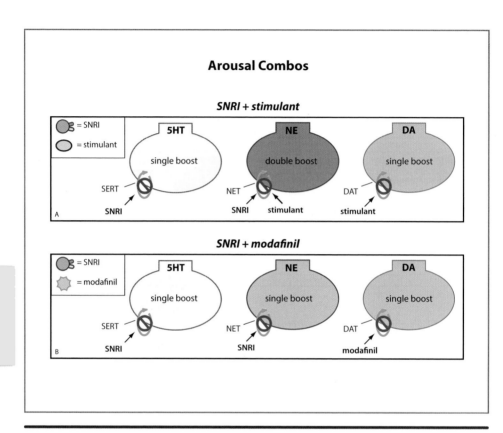

FIGURE 4.11. A) Serotonin (5HT) and dopamine (DA) are single-boosted and norepinephrine (NE) is double-boosted when a serotonin-norepinephrine reuptake inhibitor (SNRI) is combined with a stimulant. B) 5HT and NE are single-boosted by the SNRI while DA is single-boosted by modafinil (Stahl, 2021).

Switching Strategies: Second-Line Treatments for TRD

Two classes of antidepressants that are considered second-line treatments yet are rarely used today are the tricyclic antidepressants (TCAs) and the monoamine oxidase inhibitors (MAOIs).

Tricyclic antidepressants are one of the oldest classes of antidepressants and are quite efficacious; however, they are rarely prescribed now due to their unwanted side effects.

The first clinically effective drugs for depression ever discovered were inhibitors of the enzyme monoamine oxidase (MAO). While best known as powerful drugs to treat depression, they are rarely prescribed now due to dietary restrictions and drug interactions.

Tricyclic Antidepressants (TCAs)

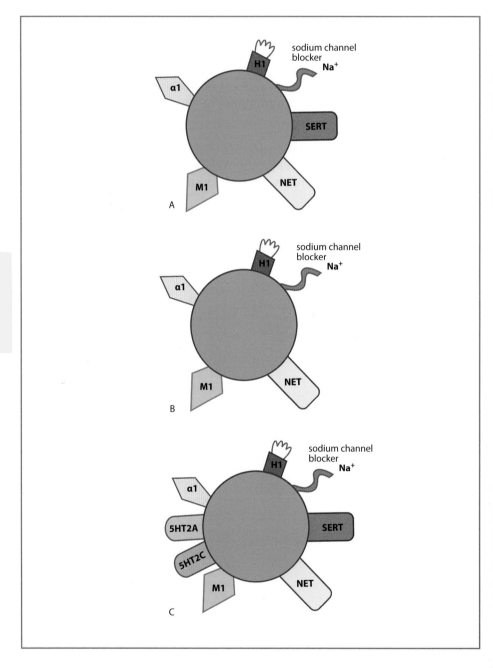

Tricyclic Antidepressants (TCAs)

FIGURE 4.12. Tricyclic antidepressants (TCAs) are quite efficacious, while rarely prescribed today. All TCAs block the reuptake of norepinephrine and are antagonists at histamine 1 (H1), α1-adrenergic and muscarinic cholinergic receptors. They also block voltage-sensitive sodium channels (A, B, and C). Additionally, some TCAs are potent inhibitors of the serotonin reuptake pump (A, C). A few are also antagonists at 5HT2A and 2C receptors (C) (Stahl, 2021). As a class, the major limitation to the TCAs has never been their efficacy, but rather that all of them share at least four other unwanted pharmacological actions, namely blockade of muscarinic cholinergic receptors, H1 histamine receptors, α1-adrenergic receptors, and voltage-sensitive sodium channels. Blockade of H1 receptors causes sedation and possible weight gain. Blocking muscarinic cholinergic receptors, also known as anticholinergic actions, causes dry mouth, blurred vision, urinary retention, and constipation. Finally, blockade of α1-adrenergic receptors, while potentially therapeutic, may result in orthostatic hypotension and dizziness. In addition, TCAs block voltage-gated sodium channels in the heart and brain. The most important of these secondary actions (at least in the event of overdose) may be the blockade of voltage-gated sodium channels because it has the potential to cause coma, seizures, cardiac arrhythmias, cardiac arrest, and even death. Nonetheless, these agents are efficacious, and they are important treatment options for patients who do not respond to first-line treatments.

Monoamine Oxidase Inhibitors

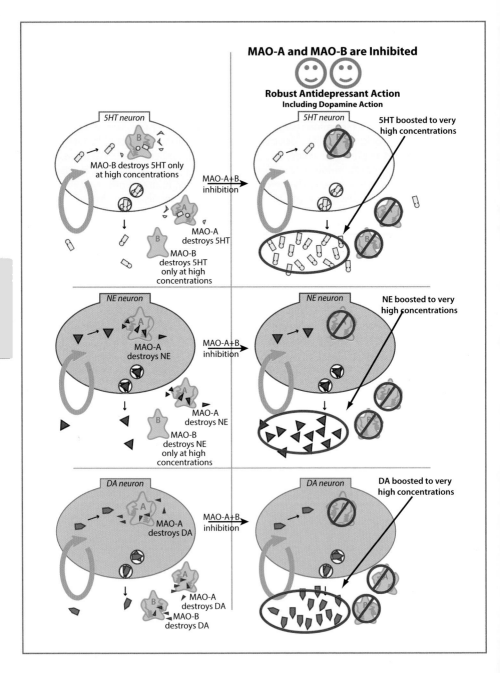

MAO-A and MAO-B are Inhibited

Robust Antidepressant Action
Including Dopamine Action

5HT neuron

MAO-B destroys 5HT only at high concentrations

MAO-A+B inhibition

MAO-A destroys 5HT

MAO-B destroys 5HT only at high concentrations

5HT neuron

5HT boosted to very high concentrations

NE neuron

MAO-A destroys NE

MAO-A+B inhibition

MAO-A destroys NE

MAO-B destroys NE only at high concentrations

NE neuron

NE boosted to very high concentrations

DA neuron

MAO-A destroys DA

MAO-A+B inhibition

MAO-A destroys DA

MAO-B destroys DA

DA neuron

DA boosted to very high concentrations

Monoamine Oxidase Inhibitors

FIGURE 4.13. Monoamine oxidase exists in two subtypes, A and B. The A form preferentially metabolizes the monoamines most closely linked to depression (serotonin and norepinephrine) whereas the B form preferentially metabolizes the trace amines such as phenethylamine. Both MAO-A and MAO-B metabolize dopamine and tyramine, another trace amine.

Brain MAO-A must be substantially inhibited for antidepressant efficacy to occur. Inhibition of MAO-B is not effective as an antidepressant, since there is no direct effect on either serotonin or norepinephrine metabolism, and little or no dopamine accumulates due to the continued action of MAO-A.

When MAO-A is inhibited simultaneously with MAO-B, there is robust elevation of dopamine as well as serotonin and norepinephrine. This would theoretically provide the most powerful antidepressant efficacy across the range of depressive symptoms, from diminished positive affect to increased negative affect. Thus, MAO-A plus MAO-B inhibition is one of the few therapeutic strategies available to increase dopamine in depression, and therefore to treat refractory symptoms of diminished positive affect (Grady and Stahl, 2015; Stahl, 2021).

Unfortunately, there are two general types of potentially dangerous interactions with MAOIs that a practitioner must be aware of: those that can raise blood pressure by sympathomimetic actions and those that can cause a potentially fatal 5HT syndrome by 5HT reuptake inhibition. Tyramine content in food can initiate a hypertensive crisis in patients taking MAOIs, where as little as 10mg of dietary tyramine can cause problems. Every patient taking MAOIs should be counseled on diet and tyramine content in foods.

Augmentation Strategies: Combine Psychotherapy With Pharmacotherapy

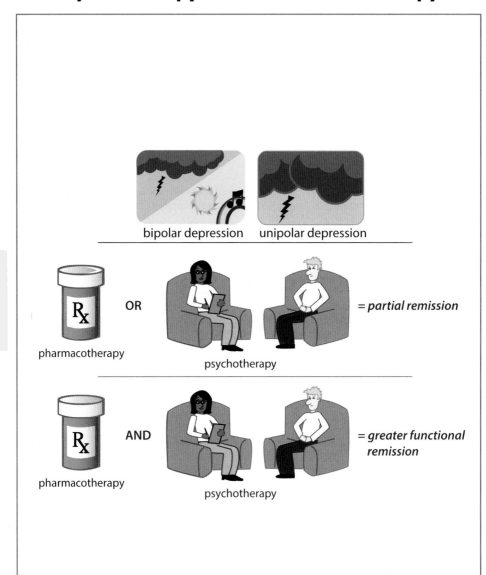

bipolar depression   unipolar depression

pharmacotherapy   OR   psychotherapy   = *partial remission*

pharmacotherapy   AND   psychotherapy   = *greater functional remission*

Augmentation Strategies: Combine Psychotherapy With Pharmacotherapy

FIGURE 4.14. Psychotherapy as an adjunct treatment to pharmacotherapy has been shown to improve overall quality of life in patients with unipolar depression and bipolar depression (van Bronswijk et al., 2019). Behavioral and educational therapies help improve factors such as total functioning, relationship functioning, life satisfaction, compliance with medication, and personal coping mechanisms. Psychotherapy can provide a necessary regular forum for patients to express and work through the progression of their illness and the coping mechanisms they use to overcome their limitations.

Augmentation Strategies:
Transcranial Magnetic Stimulation

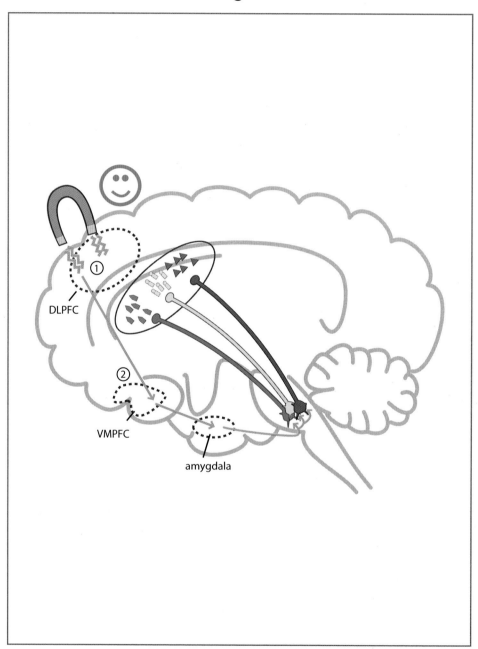

Augmentation Strategies: Transcranial Magnetic Stimulation

FIGURE 4.15. Transcranial magnetic stimulation (TMS) is a brain stimulation treatment approved for treatment-resistant depression (TRD). TMS involves placing an electromagnetic coil on the scalp, creating a magnetic field that penetrates the skull by a few centimeters and depolarizes neurons in the superficial cortex through neural pathways. This local stimulation results in functional alterations in other brain regions. The approval of TMS is based on a study of high-frequency repetitive TMS (rTMS) over the left dorsolateral prefrontal cortex (DLPFC) (O'Reardon et al., 2007), however low-frequency right side stimulation to the DLPFC has also demonstrated efficacy (Blumberger et al., 2013).

In 2013, deep TMS with an H1 coil was approved for TRD, reducing the protocol time from approximately 37 minutes to 20 minutes for 4–6 weeks. In 2018, the 3-minute theta-burst protocol was approved for TRD, shortening the time period needed to deliver treatment even further. Typical theta-burst pattern consists of three bursts of pulses at 50Hz, repeated every 200 milliseconds.

Presumably, daily stimulation of the DLPFC over several weeks causes activation of various brain circuits, leading to an antidepressant effect (Stahl, 2021). If this activates a brain circuit beginning in the DLPFC (1) and connecting to other brain areas such as the ventromedial prefrontal cortex (VMPFC) and the amygdala, with connections to the brainstem centers of the monoamine neurotransmitter system, the net result would be monoamine modulation (2). In this way, TMS could act through a mechanism unlike the known chemical antidepressants. However, TMS also releases neurotransmitters locally, in the area of the magnet, depolarizing the neurons and releasing neurotransmitters from their axon terminals in the DLPFC (1). This is a second mechanism unlike chemical antidepressants, and it may explain why TMS can still be effective in patients who do not respond to antidepressant medications.

Since all the effects of TMS are in the brain, there are no peripheral side effects such as nausea, weight gain, blood pressure changes, or sexual dysfunction. In fact, there are few, if any, side effects except headache (Berlim et al., 2013; Kalu et al., 2012).

TMS is generally done on an outpatient basis, requires no sedation or anesthesia, and does not involve loss of consciousness. The main contraindication is for patients with ferromagnetic metal within 30 cm of where the electromagnetic coil is placed. Caution should be exercised for patients with an implantable device.

Treatment-Resistant Strategies for Bipolar Depression

For years, the field has focused on effective strategies for treatment-resistant unipolar depression, however studies are lacking in science-based approaches for treatment-resistant bipolar depression. Serotonin/dopamine blocking agents originally developed for psychosis are now some of the most common adjunctive treatments to SSRIs/SNRIs in patients with unipolar depression who fail to respond adequately to one or more trials of the various first-line monoamine agents. Interestingly, this same class of drugs is often used to treat bipolar depression. Due to the different nature of depression within the context of bipolar disorder, there are many factors that contribute to medication selections for treatment (e.g., mood stabilization). Thus, strategies for treatment-resistant bipolar depression will be different than those often used for treatment-resistant unipolar depression; however, there may be overlap. In this book, we focus on evidence-based augmentation strategies: pharmacological approaches (traditional and novel strategies), brain stimulation techniques, and environmental strategies for managing treatment-resistant bipolar depression.

Augmentation Strategies:
Lithium + Lamotrigine Combination

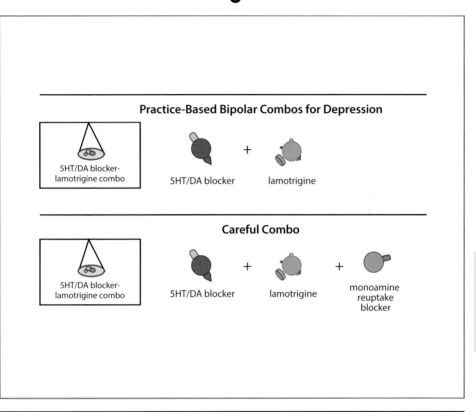

FIGURE 4.16. Most patients with bipolar disorder will require treatment with two or more agents. A combination that is not well studied in controlled trials but has practice-based evidence for bipolar depression is a serotonin/dopamine antagonist plus lamotrigine. Although controversial, some clinicians add a monoamine reuptake inhibitor to a serotonin/dopamine antagonist for bipolar depression (Stahl, 2021).

Electroconvulsive Therapy (ECT)

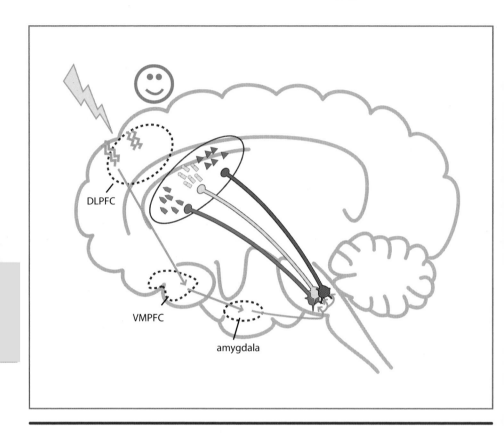

FIGURE 4.17. Electroconvulsive therapy (ECT) is a classic therapeutic form of brain stimulation for depression. It is effective in treating mania and bipolar depression. The mechanism is unknown but may be related to increased neuroplasticity following potential mobilization of neurotransmitters caused by seizure (Pittenger and Duman, 2008; Stahl, 2021). ECT has the highest rate of response and remission of any antidepressant treatment and should be considered for patients with bipolar depression or unipolar depression when they're not responsive to pharmacotherapy and psychotherapy (Gelenberg et al., 2010). ECT may be more effective than pharmacotherapy for bipolar depression (Schoeyen et al., 2015).

The best data for unipolar depression is for acute treatment. Existing data and expert clinical opinion support the idea that ECT response can be relatively rapid, often occurring after a few sessions. The acute course of ECT treatment is typically 6–12 treatments and does not generally exceed 20 treatments (Gelenberg et al., 2010). Treatment should continue until symptoms remit or plateau, as relapse rates are higher if ECT is discontinued prematurely. The most common side effect with ECT is memory loss. The frequency of sessions can affect memory loss, as patients may not have sufficient time to recover from memory effects prior to the next session (Gelenberg et al., 2010; Husain et al., 2004).

Bright Light Therapy

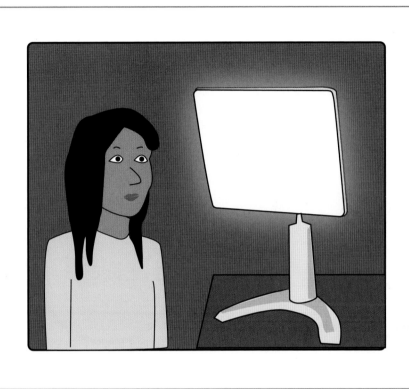

FIGURE 4.18. Light therapy is hypothesized to correct altered circadian rhythms, a condition that has been linked to depression. The clinical recommendation is for the patient to sit directly in front of the light box with 7,000–10,000 lux for 30 minutes within the first 10 minutes of waking. Studies have shown that light therapy is effective for major depressive disorder (MDD), seasonal affective disorder (SAD), and as adjunctive therapy for bipolar depression (Sit et al., 2018; Yorguner Kupeli et al., 2018; Zhou et al., 2018). At least one study has also found that sleep deprivation combined with light therapy is effective in treating bipolar depression, where total sleep deprivation plus light therapy for one week resulted in a 44% response in resistant patients (Benedetti et al., 2005); however, more research is needed. Care should be exercised in patients with bipolar disorder as there is some evidence of induction of mania.

Modafinil

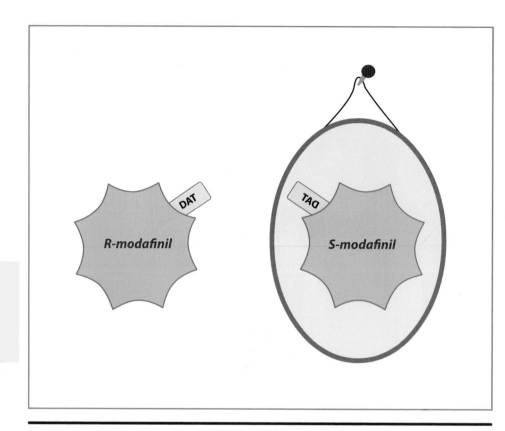

FIGURE 4.19. Modafinil consists of two enantiomers, R and S. It is primarily a weak dopamine (DA) reuptake inhibitor through its competitive binding to the cell membrane of the dopamine transporter (DAT). Additionally, modafinil binds to the norepinephrine transporter (NET), resulting in increased norepinephrine (NE). Modafinil has additional effects on several other CNS systems such as GABA, glutamate, histamine (HA), and orexin pathways (Darwish et al., 2010; He et al., 2011; Minzenberg and Carter, 2008; Morrisette, 2013). Overall, modafinil increases HA, NE, 5-HT, and DA levels in the brain (Minzenberg et al., 2008). A study in 85 patients with adjunctive modafinil (mean dosage 177mg/d) was positive without switching to mania or hypomania. Response and remission rates were higher in the modafinil group (44% and 39%) compared with the placebo group (25% and 18%) (Frye et al., 2007). However, modafinil could cause subclinical switches (Fountoulakis et al., 2008).

Ketamine

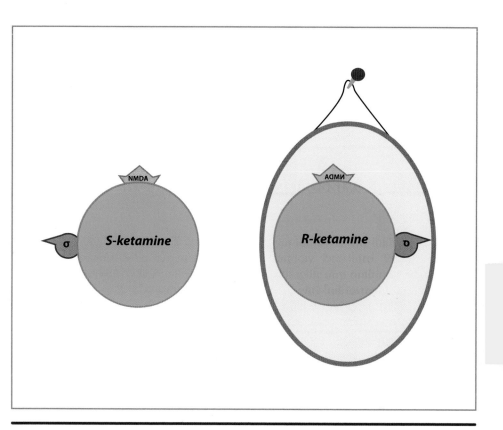

FIGURE 4.20. Ketamine has most notably had a therapeutic role in unipolar depression; however, it has also shown to be effective in treating bipolar depression as adjunctive treatment. In a systematic review of experimental studies using ketamine for the treatment of bipolar depression, data was collected from six studies (n=135) where patients were on a mood-stabilizing agent and received doses ranging from one dose to six of 0.5mg/kg intravenous racemic ketamine. The overall proportion achieving a response (defined as those having a reduction in their baseline depression severity of at least 50%) was 61% for those receiving ketamine and 5% for those receiving a placebo. The overall response rates varied from 53% to 80% across studies (Bahji et al., 2021). Two patients (one receiving ketamine and one receiving placebo) developed manic symptoms. There is also evidence that ketamine improves anxiety, agitation, and irritability in adults with treatment-resistant bipolar disorder (McIntyre et al., 2020). The preliminary evidence suggests that intravenous ketamine is effective as adjunctive treatment for bipolar depression (Zarate et al., 2012); however, further research is needed.

Chapter 5

Future Pharmacological Treatments for Depressive Disorders

In this chapter, we discuss novel treatments for depressive disorders that act through mechanisms that are not traditional for antidepressants. This includes unique receptor targets, such as glutamate, GABA, and 5HT2 receptors.

In recent years, one of the most interesting developments in the treatment of resistant unipolar depression has been the observation that infusions of subanesthetic doses of ketamine or intranasal administration of esketamine can exert immediate antidepressant effects, which was discussed earlier in this book.

Since the effects are often not sustained for more than a few days, researchers have searched for oral ketamine-like agents that could have rapid onset, sustained efficacy, and better tolerability in patients with treatment-resistant depression. Several such possibilities are in development, namely various NMDA antagonists with additional pharmacological properties, which are addressed in this chapter. We also discuss the use of hallucinogen-assisted psychotherapy, 3,4-methylene-dioxymethamphetamine (MDMA), and psilocybin.

Dextromethorphan-Bupropion and Dextromethorphan-Quinidine

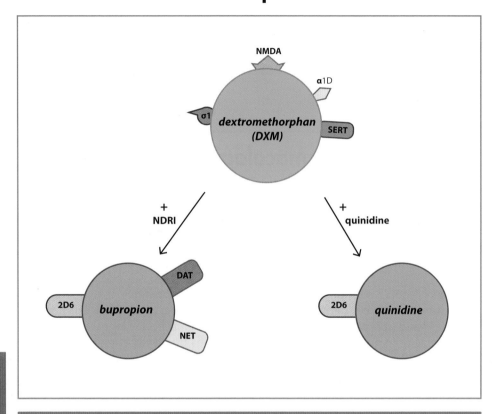

FIGURE 5.1. One agent combines the NMDA antagonist dextromethorphan with the CYP450 2D6 inhibitor and norepinephrine-dopamine reuptake inhibitor (NDRI) bupropion, and the other combines dextromethorphan with the CYP450 2D6 inhibitor quinidine. A newer version of the latter combination has deuterated the dextromethorphan molecule and altered the dose of quinidine. Deuteration extends the half-life of a compound. While it is clear that dextromethorphan has clinically relevant affinity for the NMDA receptor, other binding properties are less well characterized, including sigma-1 receptor binding, SERT inhibition, and weak μ-opioid binding (Stahl, 2013b; Stahl, 2019; Stahl, 2021). As for all NMDA receptor antagonists studied for treatment-resistant depression, it is unclear which subtypes of NMDA receptor are engaged by dextromethorphan, which are most important, and what role sigma or μ-opioid binding plays in rapid antidepressant action.

Dextromethorphan is rapidly metabolized by CYP450 2D6, making it difficult to achieve therapeutic blood levels following oral administration without concomitant administration of a CYP450 2D6 inhibitor. Quinidine is a 2D6 inhibitor at doses below its cardiovascular actions and bupropion is not only a NDRI but also a 2D6 inhibitor.

Dextromethorphan-bupropion received US FDA approval for the treatment of major depressive disorder in August of 2022.

Esmethadone

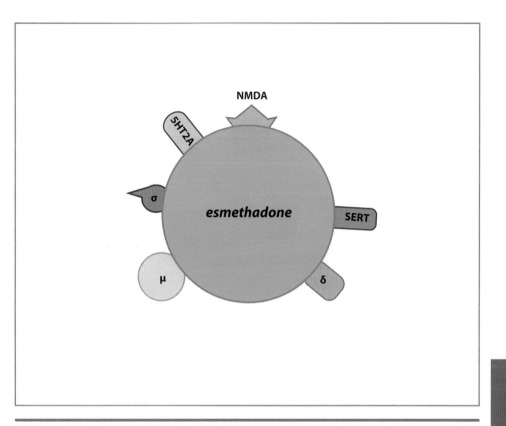

FIGURE 5.2. Methadone is a racemic mixture of S- and levomethadone and is given orally as a μ-opioid agonist for medication-assisted treatment of opioid use disorder. The μ-opioid activity resides mostly in the levo enantiomer, and the S enantiomer has relatively more potent NMDA antagonist activity, without as potent μ-opioid agonist activity. The s enantiomer is in clinical development as a rapid-onset treatment of major depression, based on positive results in animal studies (Hanania et al., 2020) with some promising early clinical results. The specific NMDA receptors targeted, and the downstream consequences of NMDA antagonism, are just now being clarified, just as for all NMDA antagonists for treatment-resistant depression (e.g., ketamine, esketamine, and dextromethorphan) (Duman and Voleti, 2012). The potential differences between these agents are also in the process of being clarified. Furthermore, the additional binding properties of each of these agents, including esmethadone, are less well characterized, such as sigma-1 receptor binding, SERT inhibition, and weak μ-opioid binding. It is possible that these agents do not act simply as NMDA antagonists, but that a certain degree of μ-opioid agonist activity may usher dimers of NMDA and μ receptors by exploiting their natural oppositional actions, to create a greater NMDA effect in the presence of μ stimulation than in the absence of it. This is the focus of much further research as the field attempts to clarify the mechanism of rapid antidepressant response associated with NMDA antagonism, and which portfolio of receptor actions is optimal.

Hallucinogen-Assisted Psychotherapy

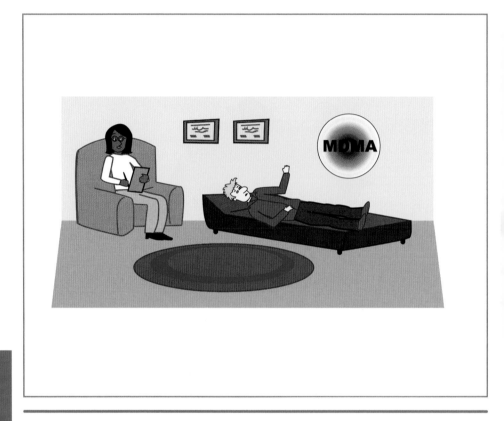

FIGURE 5.3. In the field of mental health, psychotherapy has traditionally competed with psychopharmacology. More recently, psychotherapy and psychopharmacology have come to be seen as complementary and most mental health prescribers also practice psychotherapy. Combining both psychotherapy and medication can be synergistic for many patients in terms of therapeutic efficacy and favorable long-term outcomes, perhaps by sharing some common neurobiological links, since both can alter brain circuitry. Research suggests that psychotherapy is a form of learning which can induce epigenetic changes in brain circuits, which can enhance the efficiency of information processing in malfunctioning neurons to improve symptoms in psychiatric disorders, similarly to pharmacological agents. A recent clinical exploitation of the combination of psychotherapy with psychopharmacology is a re-emergence in the use of hallucinogens to induce a dissociative state in which the patient may be more amenable to psychotherapeutic input (Carhart-Harris et al., 2016; Carhart-Harris et al., 2018). One idea is to provide more insight and clarity during this process. Another idea is to use psychotherapy-guided re-experiencing of memories, coupled with techniques to interfere with reconsolidation of traumatic memories so they are "forgotten." Animal studies show that memories are initially consolidated into relatively permanent memory files, but become labile when reactivated, and if not reconsolidated after having or modifying that memory, it can theoretically be erased (Nader et al., 2000). That is the goal of some types of hallucinogen-assisted psychotherapies: to prevent the reconsolidation of traumatic memories. Several agents have been tested in this paradigm of dissociation-assisted psychotherapy, from ketamine to MDMA and psilocybin.

3,4-Methylene-Dioxymethamphetamine (MDMA)

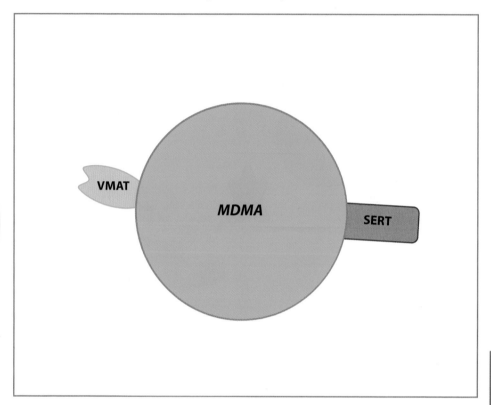

FIGURE 5.4. 3,4-Methylene-dioxymethamphetamine (MDMA) is an amphetamine derivative that transforms amphetamine itself from being predominantly a norepinephrine-dopamine reuptake inhibitor with vesicular monoamine transporter 2 (VMAT2) inhibition causing enhanced dopamine release into a more powerful serotonin reuptake inhibitor with VMAT2 inhibition causing increased serotonin release as well. The released serotonin is free to act at all serotonin receptors but seems to have profound actions in stimulating the 5HT2A receptor, not unlike other hallucinogens. MDMA may be helpful in psychotherapy because it can produce feelings of increased energy, pleasure, and emotional warmth, promoting trust and closeness. However, it also causes distortions and hallucinations of sensory and time perception. Its 5HT2A agonist actions may be responsible for the spike in body temperature that can occur after taking MDMA, with organ damage and even death, especially when dancing all night and when dehydrated. MDMA found on the streets is often contaminated with "bath salts" (synthetic cathinones), methamphetamine, dextromethorphan, ketamine, and/or cocaine and is often consumed with marijuana and alcohol. Pure MDMA is what is studied in hallucinogen-assisted psychotherapy. MDMA is in testing for PTSD, anxiety, and existential distress in terminally ill patients, social anxiety in autism, treatment refractory depression, substance abuse, and more (Reiff et al., 2020; Stahl, 2021).

Psilocybin
4-phosphoryloxy-N,N-dimethyltryptamine

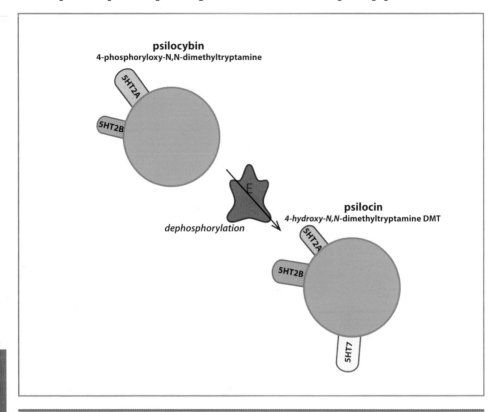

FIGURE 5.5. Psilocybin (4-phosphoryloxy-N, N-dimethyltryptamine), also known as a hallucinogen in "magic mushrooms," has a structure similar to lysergic acid diethylamide (LSD) and has been used and abused for its ability to cause hallucinogenic, psychedelic, and euphoric "trips." Psilocybin is rapidly converted to its active metabolite psilocin (4-hydroxy-N,N-dimethyltryptamine or DMT) by dephosphorylation. Both agents bind to a number of serotonin receptor subtypes (5HT1A, 5HT2A, 5HT2C, and others), but the hallucinogenic actions of both agents are linked most closely with agonist actions on 5HT2A receptors, since 5HT2A antagonists (but not selective dopamine D2 antagonists) reverse the effects of psilocybin in humans. Studies suggest that psilocybin combined with psychotherapy is effective for treatment-resistant depression (Carhart-Harris et al., 2016; Carhart-Harris et al., 2018). Psilocybin has been designated as a breakthrough therapy by the United States Food and Drug Administration (US FDA) for the treatment of depression. Psilocybin is also being widely investigated for anxiety and existential distress in terminally ill patients, substance abuse, PTSD, and several other conditions.

Nonpharmacological Treatments for Depressive Disorders

In Chapter 6, we discuss nonpharmacological approaches for treating depressive disorders. The majority of these strategies have been utilized as adjunctive treatments. However, they may be used alone when pharmacological approaches have not been effective or when there is resistance to pharmacological treatment. Psychotherapy, bright light therapy, exercise, and brain stimulation techniques such as transcranial magnetic stimulation (TMS) and electroconvulsive therapy (ECT) will be discussed.

Psychotherapy

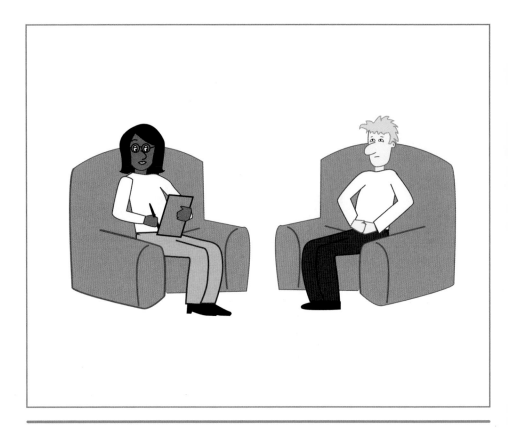

FIGURE 6.1. Psychotherapy can be an effective form of treatment for depressive disorders, however it's not typically recommended as first-line treatment. In a recent meta-analysis, psychotherapy alone was not superior to treatment as usual (TAU) for depression. TAU was defined as continued management of or optimization of pharmacotherapy for depression (van Bronswijk et al., 2019). When psychotherapy was added to TAU it was effective as adjunctive treatment for depression (van Bronswijk et al., 2019). Psychotherapy includes a variety of formats, including cognitive behavioral therapy (CBT), psychoanalytic applications, and others.

Bright Light Therapy

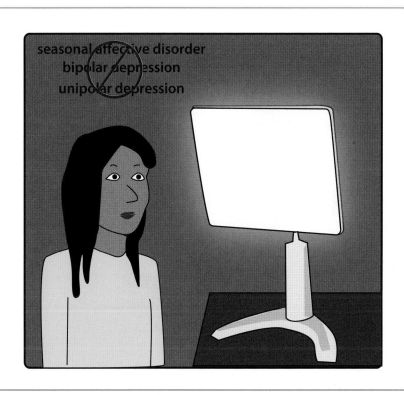

FIGURE 6.2. For over three decades bright light therapy (BLT) has been used to treat seasonal affective disorder (SAD), unipolar depression, and bipolar depression, with a growing body of literature to support its efficacy. BLT has physiological effects by resynchronizing the biological clock (circadian system), enhancing alertness, increasing sleep pressure (homeostatic system), and acting on serotonin and other monoaminergic pathways. Side effects may be nausea, diarrhea, headache, and eye irritation, and are generally mild and rare. A recent review suggests that BLT is an efficient antidepressant strategy in mono- or adjunct therapy that should be personalized according to the unipolar or bipolar subtype, the presence or absence of seasonal patterns, and also regarding its efficacy and tolerability (Maruani and Geoffroy, 2019).

Brain Stimulation Techniques

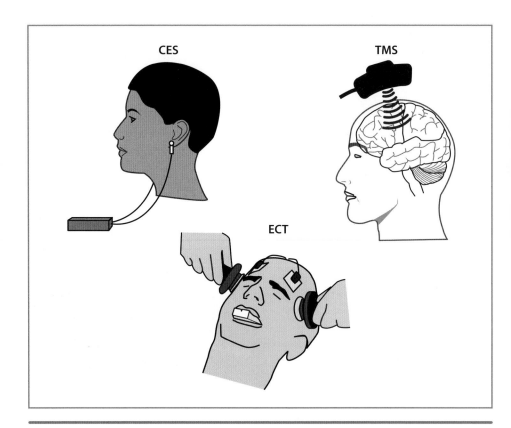

FIGURE 6.3. A variety of brain stimulation techniques have been used since the late 1930s to treat depressive disorders. Electroconvulsive therapy (ECT) is the oldest form of brain stimulation and still to this day has the highest response/remission rates of any depression treatment. Remission rates after one round of ECT were 51.5% for unipolar depression and 50.9% for bipolar depression (Jevolac et al., 2013; Kellner et al., 2006; Micallef-Trigona, 2014; Sackeim et al., 2001; Sackeim et al., 2009). Unfortunately, relapse rates are also high, particularly if used as monotherapy, and there are unwanted side effects (e.g., memory loss). Cranial electrotherapy (CES) is FDA-approved for depression, insomnia, and anxiety. Electrodes are placed on the ear lobes, maxilla-occipital junction, mastoid processes, or temples, and CES stimulation induces alterations in EEG waves (e.g., it increases alpha relative power and decreases delta and beta frequencies) (Kirsch and Nichols, 2013). Transcranial magnetic stimulation (TMS) was approved as adjunctive treatment for depression in 2008; however, it is now used off-label as monotherapy and to treat a variety of other mental health conditions. There are many variations: repetitive TMS (rTMS), deep TMS, and theta-burst rTMS, which involve various types of coils and protocols. Other brain stimulation techniques worth noting are transcranial direct current stimulation (tDCS) and trigeminal nerve stimulation (TNS).

Exercise

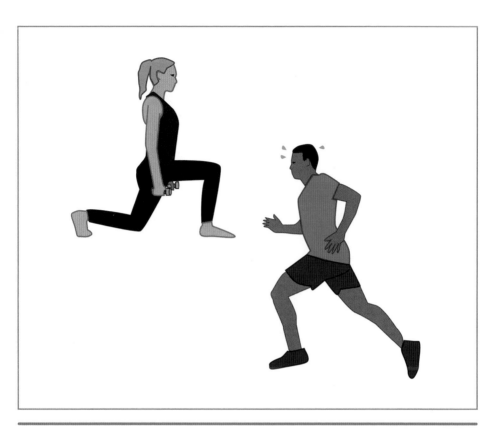

FIGURE 6.4. Exercise may be effective as monotherapy or adjunctive therapy for the treatment of depression. A meta-analysis suggests that physical activity can help prevent the onset and relapse of depression (Andersson et al., 2015). Patients with depression are encouraged to engage in aerobic exercise and/or muscular strength training. There is strong evidence that physical activity alone is beneficial for the treatment of mild and moderate depression and can reduce symptoms of mild to moderate depression to the same extent as standard treatments (psychotherapy and antidepressant medication) (Andersson et al., 2015). There are a variety of theories as to potential mechanisms that underlie the benefits of exercise for mental health. These include improved mitochondria function, enhanced mammalian target of rapamycin (mTOR) signaling, alterations in monoamines (e.g., serotonin and norepinephrine), reduced inflammation, increased vagal tone, enhanced neuroplasticity, and increased neurogenesis. Combining exercise with psychotherapy and antidepressant medication may yield additional benefits (Andersson et al., 2015).

Stahl's Illustrated | Summary

As our understanding of the neurobiological and molecular bases of mood disorders expands, it is becoming increasingly obvious that malfunctioning circuits underlie the specific symptoms that need treatment. When mood disorders are viewed as part of a spectrum, this allows for earlier and more accurate diagnoses, resulting in optimal treatment and management of symptoms. Finally, a deeper understanding of the mechanisms that underlie disrupted neurocircuitry in mood disorders will allow for further advancement of novel therapeutic targets in pharmacological treatments, resulting in better outcomes for patients.

Stahl's Illustrated | References

Aan het Rot M, Collins KA, Murrough JW et al. Safety and efficacy of repeated-dose intravenous ketamine for treatment-resistant depression. Biol Psychiatry 2010;67:139-45.

Alvarez LD, Pecci A, Estrin DA. In search of GABA A receptor's neurosteroid binding sites. J Med Chem 2019;62:5250-60.

American Psychiatric Association. Diagnostic and statistical manual of mental disorders, fifth edition, text revision. Washington, DC: American Psychiatric Publishing; 2022.

Andersson E, Hovland A, Kjellman B et al. Physical activity just as good as CBT or drugs for depression. Lakartidningen 2015;112:DP4E.

Artigas F. Serotonin receptors involved in antidepressant effects. Pharmacol Ther 2013;137:119-31.

Bahji A, Zarate CA, Vazquez GH. Ketamine for bipolar depression: a systematic review. Int J Neuropsychopharmacol 2021;24(7):535-41.

Belelli D, Hogenkamp D, Gee KW et al. Realizing the therapeutic potential of neuroactive steroid modulators of the GABA A receptor. Neurobiol Stress 2020;12:100207.

Benedetti F, Barbini B, Fulgosi MC et al. Combined total sleep deprivation and light therapy in the treatment of drug-resistant bipolar depression: acute response and long-term remission rates. J Clin Psychiatry 2005;66:1535-40.

Berlim MT, Van den Eynde F, Daskalakis ZJ. Clinically meaningful efficacy and acceptability of low-frequency repetitive transcranial magnetic stimulation (rTMS) for treating primary major depression: a meta-analysis of randomized, double-blind, and sham-controlled trials. Neuropsychopharmacology 2013;38:543-51.

Blumberger DM, Mulsant BH, Daskalakis ZJ. What is the role of brain stimulation therapies in the treatment of depression? Curr Psychiatry Rep 2013;15(7):368.

Bostwick JM. A generalist's guide to treating patients with depression with an emphasis on using side effects to tailor antidepressant therapy. Mayo Clin Proc 2010;85(6):538-50.

Botella GM, Salitur FG, Harrison BL et al. Neuroactive steroids. 2. 3α-hydroxy, 3β-methyl-21-(4-cyano-1H-pyrazol-1'-yl)-19-nor-5β-pregnan-20-one (SAGE 217): a clinical next generation neuroactive steroid positive allosteric modulator of the (γ-aminobutyric acid) A receptor. J Med Chem 2017;60:7810-19.

Brites D, Fernandes A. Neuroinflammation and depression: microglia activation, extracellular microvesicles and microRNA dysregulation. Front Cell Neurosci 2015;9(476):1-20.

Carhart-Harris RL, Bolstridge M, Day CMG et al. Psilocybin with psychological support for treatment-resistant depression: six-month follow-up. Psychopharmacology 2018;235:399-408.

Carhart-Harris RL, Bolstridge M, Rucker J et al. Psilocybin with psychological support for treatment-resistant depression: an open-label feasibility study. Lancet Psychiatry 2016;3:619-27.

Carr GV, Lucki I. The role of serotonin receptor subtypes in treating depression: review of animal studies. Psychopharmacology (Berl) 2011;213(2-3):265-87.

Cascade E, Kalali AH, Kennedy SH. Real-world data on SSRI antidepressant side effects. Psychiatry (Edgmont) 2009;6(2):16-18.

Chen ZW, Braomonies JR, Budelier MM et al. Multiple functional neurosteroid binding sites on GABAA receptors. PLOS Biol 2019;17:e3000157.

Chiu CT, Chuang DM. Molecular actions and therapeutic potential of lithium in preclinical and clinical studies of CNS disorder. Pharmacol Ther 2010;128:281-304.

Conradi HJ, Ormel J, Jonge PD. Presence of individual (residual) symptoms during depressive episodes and periods of remission: a 3-year prospective study. Psychol Med 2011;41(6):1165-74.

Darwish M, Kirby M, D'Andrea DM et al. Pharmacokinetics of armodafinil and modafinil after single and multiple doses in patients with excessive sleepiness associated with treated obstructive sleep apnea: a randomized, open-label, crossover study. Clin Ther 2010;32(12):2074-87.

Dowlati Y, Herrmann N, Swardfager W et al. A meta-analysis of cytokines in major depression. Biol Psychiatry 2010;67:446-7.

Duffy FF, Chung H, Trivedi M et al. Systematic use of patient-related depression severity monitoring: is it helpful and feasible in clinical psychiatry? Psychiatr Serv 2008;59(10):1148-54.

Duman RS, Voleti B. Signaling pathways underlying the pathophysiology and treatment of depression: novel mechanisms for rapid-acting agents. Trends Neurosci 2012;35:47-56.

Fiedorowicz JG, Endicott J, Leon AC et al. Subthreshold hypomanic symptoms in progression from unipolar major depression to bipolar disorder. Am J Psychiatry 2011;168:40-8.

Fink KB, Gothert M. 5-HT receptor regulation of neurotransmitter release. Pharmacol Rev 2007;59(4):360-417.

Fountoulakis KN, Siamouli M, Panagiotidis P et al. Ultra short manic-like episodes after antidepressant augmentation with modafinil. Prog Neuropsychopharmacol Biol Psychiatry 2008;32(3):891-2.

Frye MA, Grunze H, Suppes T et al. A placebo-controlled evaluation of adjunctive modafinil in the treatment of bipolar depression. Am J Psychiatry 2007;164:1242-9.

Gartlehner R, Hansen RA, Carey TS et al. Discontinuation rates for selective serotonin reuptake inhibitors and other second-generation antidepressants in outpatients with major depressive disorder: a systematic review and meta-analysis. Int Clin Psychopharmacol 2005;20:59-69.

Gelenberg AJ. A review of the current guidelines for depression treatment. J Clin Psychiatry 2010;71(7):e15.

Gerrard, P Malcom R. Mechanisms of modafinil: a review of current research. Neuropsychiatric Disease and Treatment 2007;3(3): 349–64

Giovanni MG, Ceccarelli I, Molinari B et al. Serotonergic modulation of acetylcholine release from cortex of freely moving rats. J Pharmacol Exp Ther 1998;285(3):1219-25.

Grady M, Stahl SM. The road to remission: optimizing pharmacological treatment of unipolar depression. New York, NY: Cambridge University Press; 2015.

Hanania T, Manfredi P, Inturrisi C et al. The N-methyl-D-aspartate receptor antagonist d-methadone acutely improves depressive-like behavior in the forced swim test performance of rats. Exp Clin Psychopharmacol 2020;28(2):196-201.

Harshing LG Jr, Prauda I, Brakoczy J et al. A 5-HT7 heteroreceptor-mediated inhibition of [3H] serotonin release in raphe nuclei slices of the rat: evidence for a serotonergic-glutamatergic interaction. Neurochem Res 2004;29(8):1487-97.

He B, Peng H, Zhao Y et al. Modafinil treatment prevents REM sleep deprivation-induced brain function impairment by increasing MMP-9-expression. Brain Res 2011;1426:28-32.

Henssler J, Alexander D, Schwarzer G et al. Combining antidepressants vs antidepressant monotherapy for treatment of patients with acute depression: a systematic review and meta-analysis. JAMA Psychiatry 2022;79(4):300-12.

Howren MB, Lamkin DM, Suls J. Associations of depression with c-reactive protein IL-1 and IL-6: a meta-analysis. Psychosom Med 2009; 71:171-86.

Husain MM, Rush AJ, Fink M et al. Speed of response and remission in major depressive disorder with acute electroconvulsive therapy (ECT): a consortium for research in ECT (CORE) report. J Clin Psychiatry 2004;65(4):485-91.

Ibrahim L, Diaz Granados N, Franco-Chaves J. Course of improvement in depressive symptoms to a single intravenous infusion of ketamine vs. add-on riluzole: results from a 4-week, double-blind, placebo-controlled study. Neuropsychopharmacology 2012;37:1526-33.

Jevolac A, Kolshus E, McLoughlin DM. Relapse following successful electroconvulsive therapy for major depression: a meta-analysis. Neuropsychopharmacology 2013;38(12):2467-74.

Judd LL, Akiskal HS, Maser JD, et al. Major depressive disorder: a prospective study of residual subthreshold depressive symptoms as predictor of rapid relapse. J Affect Disord 1998;50(2-3):97-108.

Kalu UG, Sexton CE, Loo CK et al. Transcranial direct current stimulation in the treatment of major depression: a meta-analysis. Psychological Med 2012;42(9):1791-800.

Keller J, Gomez R, Williams G et al. HPA axis in major depression: cortisol, clinical symptomatology, and genetic variation predict cognition. Mol Psychiatry 2017;22(4):527-36.

Kellner CH, Knapp RG, Petrides G et al. Continuation electroconvulsive therapy vs pharmacotherapy for relapse prevention in major depression: a multisite study from the consortium for research in electroconvulsive therapy (CORE). Arch Gen Psychiatry 2006;63(12):1337-44.

Kelly K, Posternak M, Alpert JE. Toward achieving optimal response: understanding and managing antidepressant side effects. Dialogues Clin Neurosci 2008;10(4):109-18.

Kessler, RC, Merikangas KR, Wang PS. Prevalence, comorbidity, and service utilization for mood disorders in the United States at the beginning of the twenty-first century. 2007 In S Nolen-Hoeksema, T. Cannon & Widiger (Eds.), Ann Rev Clin Psychol 2007;3:137-58.

Kirsch DL, Nichols F. Cranial electrotherapy stimulation for treatment of anxiety, depression, and insomnia. Psychiatr Clin North Am 2013;36(1):169-76.

Kohler S, Cirpinsky K, Kronenberg G et al. The serotonergic system in the neurobiology of depression: relevance for novel antidepressants. J Psychopharmacol 2016;30(1):13-22.

Kubota Y. Untangling GABAergic wiring in the cortical microcircuit. Curr Opin Neurobiol 2014;26:7-14.

Li N, Lee B, Lin RJ et al. mTor-dependent synapse formation underlies the rapid antidepressant effects of NMDA antagonists. Science 2010;329:959-64.

Little A. Treatment-resistant depression. Am Fam Physician 2009;80(2):167-72.

Lorenz TA, Meston CM. Exercise improves sexual function in women taking antidepressants: results from a randomized crossover trial. Depress Anxiety 2014;31:188-95.

Lüscher B, Möhler H. Brexanolone, a neurosteroid antidepressant, vindicates the GABAergic deficit hypothesis of depression and may foster reliance. F1000Res 2019;8:751.

Mann JJ. The serotonergic system in mood disorders and suicidal behavior. Philos Trans R Soc Lond B Biol Sci 2013;368(1615):20120537.

Maruani J, Geoffroy PA. Bright light as a personalized treatment of mood disorders. Front Psychiatry 2019;10(85):1-9.

McIntyre RS, Durgam S, Huo J et al. The efficacy of lumateperone in patients with bipolar depression with and without mixed features. Eur Neuropsychopharmacol 2021;53(suppl 1):S305.

McIntyre RS, Lipsitz O, Rodrigues NB et al. The effectiveness of ketamine on anxiety, irritability, and agitation: Implications for treating mixed features in adults with major depressive or bipolar disorder. Bipolar Disord 2020;22:831.

Meltzer-Brody S, Kanes SJ. Allopregnanolone in postpartum depression: role in pathophysiology and treatment. Neurobiol Stress 2020;12:100212.

Micallef-Trigona B. Comparing the effects of repetitive transcranial magnetic stimulation and electroconvulsive therapy in the treatment of depression: a systematic review and meta-analysis. Depress Res Treat 2014;2014:1-8.

Miller AH, Maletic V, Raison CL. Inflammation and its discontents: the role of cytokines in the pathophysiology of major depression. Biol Psychiatry 2009;65(9):732-41.

Minzenberg MJ, Carter CS. Modafinil: a review of neurochemical actions and effects on cognition. Neuropsychopharmacology 2008;33(7):1477-502.

Morehouse R, Macqueen G, Kennedy SH. Barriers to achieving treatment goals: a focus on sleep disturbance and sexual dysfunction. J Affective Disord 2011;132:S14-20.

Morrisette DA. Twisting the night away. A review of the neurobiology, genetics, diagnosis, and treatment of shift work disorder. CNS Spectrums 2013;18(suppl 1):45-53.

Murrough JW, Perez AM, Pillemer S et al. Rapid and longer-term antidepressant effects of repeated ketamine infusions in treatment resistant major depression. Biol Psychiatry 2013;74:250-6.

Nader K, Schafe GE, Le Doux JE. Fear memories require protein synthesis in the amygdala for reconsolidation after retrieval. Nature 2000;406(6797):722-6.

Ohno Y, Shimizu S, Tokudome K. Pathophysiological roles of serotonergic system in regulating extrapyramidal motor functions. Biol Pharm Bull 2013;36(9):1396-400.

O'Reardon JP, Solvason HB, Janicak PG et al. Efficacy and safety of transcranial magnetic stimulation in the acute treatment of major depression: a multisite randomized controlled trial. Biol Psychiatry 2007;62(11):1208-16.

Pace TW, Hu F, Miller AH. Cytokine-effects on glucocorticoid receptor function: relevance to glucocorticoid resistance and the pathophysiology and treatment of major depression. Brain Behav Immun 2007;21:9-19.

Pariante CM. Risk factors for development of depression and psychosis. Glucocorticoid receptors and pituitary implications for treatment with antidepressant and glucocorticoids. Ann NY Acad Sci 2009;1179:144-52.

Pittenger C, Duman RS. Stress, depression, and neuroplasticity: a convergence of mechanisms. Neuropsychopharmacology 2008;33(I):88-109.

Puig MV, Watakabe A, Ushimaru M, et al. Serotonin modulates fast-spiking interneuron and synchronous activity in the rat prefrontal cortex through 5-HT1A and 5-HT2A receptors. J Neurosci 2010;30(6):2211-22.

Raskin J, Wiltse CG, Siegal A, et al. Efficacy of duloxetine on cognition, depression, and pain in elderly patients with major depressive disorder: an 8-week, double-blind, placebo-controlled trial. Am J Psychiatry 2007;164(6):900-909.

Reiff CM, Richman EE, Nemeroff CB et al. Psychedelics and psychedelic-assisted psychotherapy. Am J Psychiatry 2020;177(5):391-410.

Rost K. Disability from depression: the public health challenge to primary care. Nord J Psychiatry 2009;63:17-21.

Rush AJ, Trivedi MH, Wisniewski SR et al. Acute and longer-term outcomes in depressed outpatients requiring one or several treatment steps: a STAR*D report. Am J Psychiatry 2006;163(II):1905-17.

Sackeim HA, Dillingham EM, Prudic J et al. Effect of concomitant pharmacotherapy on electroconvulsive therapy outcomes: short-term efficacy and adverse effects. Arch Gen Psychiatry 2009;66(7):729-37.

Sackeim HA, Haskett RF, Mulsant BH et al. Continuation pharmacotherapy in the prevention of relapse following electroconvulsive therapy: a randomized controlled trial. JAMA 2001;285(10):1299-307.

Sage Therapeutics, Inc., "Sage Therapeutics and Biogen Announce the Phase 3 Coral Study Met Its Primary and Key Secondary Endpoints - Comparing Zuranolone 50 Mg Co-Initiated with Standard of Care Antidepressant vs. Standard of Care Co-Initiated with Placebo in People with MDD." February 16, 2022. https://investor.sagerx.com/news-releases/news-release-details/sage-therapeutics-and-biogen-announce-phase-3-coral-study-met.

SAMHSA, Center for Behavioral Health Statistics and Quality. "Key Substance Use and Mental Health Indicators in the United States: Results from the 2020 National Survey on Drug Use and Health." www.samhsa.gov/data/sites/default/files/reports/rpt35319/2020NSDUHFFR102121.htm.

Sarkisyan G, Roberts AJ, Hedlund PB. The 5-HT(7) receptor as a mediator and modulator of antidepressant-like behavior. Behav Brain Res 2010;209(1):99-108.

Satyanarayanan S, Su H, Lin Y et al. Circadian rhythm and melatonin in the treatment of depression. Curr Pharm Des 2018;24(22):2549-55.

Saveanu R, Etkin A, Duchemin AM et al. The international study to predict optimized treatment in depression (iSPOT-D): outcomes from the acute phase of antidepressant treatment. J Psychiatr Res 2015;61:1-12.

Schoeyen HK, Kessler U, Andreassen OA et al. Treatment-resistant bipolar depression: a randomized controlled trial of electroconvulsive therapy versus algorithm-based pharmacological treatment. Am J Psychiatry 2015;172(1):41-51.

Schwartz TL, Siddiqui US, Stahl SM. Vilazodone: a brief pharmacologic and clinical review of the novel SPARI (serotonin partial agonist and reuptake inhibitor). Ther Adv Psychopharmacol 2011;1:81-7.

Settimo L, Taylor D. Evaluating the dose-dependent mechanism of action of trazodone by estimation of occupancies for different brain neurotransmitter targets. J Psychopharmacol 2018;32:960104.

Sit DK, McGowan J, Wiltrout C et al. Adjunctive bright light therapy for bipolar depression: a randomized double-blind placebo-controlled trial. Am J Psychiatry 2018;175:131-9.

Srikiatkhachorn A. Pathophysiology of chronic daily headache. Curr Pain Headache Rep 2001;5(6):537-44.

Stahl SM. Mechanism of action of ketamine. CNS Spectrums 2013a;18:225-7.

Stahl SM. Mechanism of action of dextromethorphan/quinidine: comparison with ketamine. CNS Spectrums 2013b;18:225-7.

Stahl SM. Mechanism of action of the SPARI vilazodone: (serotonin partial agonist reuptake inhibitor). CNS Spectrums 2014a;19:105-9.

Stahl SM. Mechanism of action of agomelatine: a novel antidepressant exploiting synergy between monoaminergic and melatonergic properties. CNS Spectrums 2014b;19:207-12.

Stahl SM. Modes and nodes explain the mechanism of action of vortioxetine, multimodal agent (MMA): enhancing serotonin release by combining serotonin (5HT) transporter inhibition with actions at 5HT receptors (5HT1A, 5HT1B, 5HT1D, 5HT7 receptors). CNS Spectrums 2015a;20:93-7.

Stahl SM. Modes and nodes explain the mechanism of action of vortioxetine, multimodal agent (MMA): actions at serotonin receptors may enhance downstream release of four pro-cognitive neurotransmitters. CNS Spectrums 2015b;20:515-19.

Stahl SM. Drugs for psychosis and mood: unique actions at D3, D2, and D1 dopamine receptor subtypes. CNS Spectrums 2017;22:375-84.

Stahl SM. Mechanism of action of dextromethorphan/bupropion: a novel NMDA antagonist with multimodal activity. CNS Spectrums 2019;24:461-6.

Stahl SM. Stahl's essential psychopharmacology: neuroscientific basis and practical applications. 5th ed. New York, NY: Cambridge University Press; 2021.

Stahl SM, Morrisette DA. Mixed mood states: baffled, bewildered, befuddled, and bemused. Bipolar Disord 2019;21:560-1.

Stahl SM, Fava M, Trivedi MH et al. Agomelatine in the treatment of major depressive disorder: an 8-week, multicenter, randomized, placebo-controlled trial. J Clin Psychiatry 2010;71:616-26.

Stahl SM, Laredo SA, Morrisette DA. Cariprazine as a treatment across the bipolar I spectrum from depression to mania: mechanism of action and review of clinical data. Ther Adv Psychopharmacol 2020;10:1-11.

Suppes T, Silva R, Cuccharino J et al. Lurasidone for the treatment of major depressive disorder with mixed features: a randomized, double-blind placebo-controlled study. Am J Psychiatry 2016;173:400-7.

Trivedi MH. Tools and strategies for ongoing assessment of depression: a measurement-based approach to remission. J Clin Psychiatry 2009;70 (suppl 6):26-31.

van Bronswijk S, Moopen N, Beijers L, Ruhe HG, Peeters F. Effectiveness of psychotherapy for treatment-resistant depression: a meta-analysis and meta-regression. Psychol Med 2019;49(3):366-79.

Vavakova M, Durackova Z, Trebaticka J. Markers of oxidative stress and neuroprogression in depression disorder. Oxid Med Cell Longev 2015;2015:898393.

Wajs E, Aluisio L, Holder R et al. Esketamine nasal spray plus oral antidepressant in patients with treatment-resistant depression: assessment of long-term safety in a phase 3 open-label study (SUSTAIN2). J Clin Psychiatry 2020;81:19m12891.

Yorguner Kupeli N, Bulut NS, Carkaxhiu Bulut G, Kurt E, Kora K. Efficacy of bright light therapy in bipolar depression. Psychiatry Res 2018;260:432-8.

Zajecka J, Schatzberg A, Stahl SM et al. Efficacy and safety of agomelatine in the treatment of major depressive disorder: a multicenter, randomized, double-blind, placebo-controlled trial. J Clin Psychopharmacol 2010;30:135-44.

Zarate CA Jr., Brutsche NE, Ibrahim L. Replication of ketamine's antidepressant efficacy in bipolar depression: a randomized controlled add-on trial. Biol Psychiatry 2012;71:939-46.

Zhang L, Hendrick JP. The presynaptic D2 partial agonist lumateperone acts as a postsynaptic D2 antagonist. Matters 2018;doi:10.19185/matters.201712000006.

Zhou TH, Dang WM, Ma YT et al. Clinical efficacy, onset time, and safety of bright light therapy in acute bipolar depression as an adjunctive therapy: a randomized controlled trial. J Affect Disord 2018;227:90-6.